CONTENTS

B

You might well find yourself in a situation where you need to give the impression that you've been there, done it, got the T-shirt, suffered the blisters … and that there is nothing that anybody can teach you about the noble art of walking.

THE PATH OF ENLIGHTENMENT

Mankind has been walking since around 3 million years BC (Before Cars), so understandably, human feet are probably in need of a rest. That is largely why the internal combustion engine was invented.

However, after a century or so of increasing reliance on mechanised transport methods, some people prefer to leave these behind and still strike out on Shanks's pony (*see* Glossary, page 125). This is mainly because, in today's congested world, it's generally quicker.

Bluffers should be aware that hikers come in many shades, which include the following:

Ambler Someone who is not in a hurry.
Rambler Someone interested in just wandering around while talking at the same time.
Walker Someone keen on getting from A to B.
Nordic walker Someone keen on getting from A to B

energetically, by swinging their arms and shoulders and using long, pointy sticks.

Speed-walker Someone who wants to get from A to B before the bus does.

Hiker A dedicated walker whose aim in life is to tramp trails, fill his or her lungs with fresh air, yodel in the foothills and be at one with nature.

Hitch-hiker A hiker who cheats.

Hiking for enjoyment, otherwise known as walking for the sheer pleasure of it, has several benefits. Not only is the physical exercise an excellent way to maintain an ideal body weight, but it also releases endorphins, natural chemicals that make one feel calmer, happier and more relaxed.

Until, of course, you realise that you've just taken a wrong turn.

Hiking has benefits other than for health. It allows you to see aspects of the world that those sitting in cars miss as they speed past: perhaps a buzzard soaring on a thermal of warm air, a rabbit darting across the path, a red admiral warming its wings in the sun, a raptor tearing apart a small, furry animal – whereas the only wildlife motorists see is generally roadkill, and one squishy mess looks just like any other.

The path to physical fitness, mental stimulation and creative inspiration therefore means donning the right boots, selecting the right map, aiming towards the right pub, and taking the path of righteous enlightenment – one measured step at a time.

But why would you want to bluff about hiking in

the first place? Because you might well find yourself in a situation where you need to give the impression that you've been there, done it, got the T-shirt, suffered the blisters … and that there is nothing that anybody can teach you about the noble art of walking. Then, even if the limit of your knowledge is that it involves putting one foot in front of the other and propelling yourself in a roughly forwards direction (unless you're retracing your steps – something hikers do a lot), you'll need to look no further than this book as the ultimate source of all you need to know to persuade others that you're a hiker of rare ability and experience.

And it will do more. It will give you the key to the ultimate bluff: how to impress legions of marvelling listeners with your wisdom and advice, without anybody discovering that you can't find your way to the local bus stop.

Just hope they don't follow you.

Never ask another hiker for directions. Not only does it confirm that you're utterly clueless, but for all you know, he or she may also be temporarily misplaced.

GETTING YOUR BEARINGS

The art of getting lost is a well-practised one, and it is made easier today with the use of maps and other satellite navigation aids.

Of course, a real hiker is never, ever lost – merely 'temporarily misplaced'.

If you find yourself in such a situation and a fellow walker approaches, it is best to scrutinise your map closely and then, just as the walker comes within earshot, say 'Aha!' loudly and clearly, and tap your finger on the map before folding it up and walking in the opposite direction from your fellow hiker.

Never ask another hiker for directions. Not only does it confirm that you're utterly clueless, but for all you know, he or she may also be temporarily misplaced.

SYMBOLS

Bluffers who have never examined a map closely before may find the experience daunting. There's no need to worry, though, because every map comes with its own key to unlock the mystery.

If you're just stepping out, the important symbols to look out for are:

Green dotted or dashed lines These are footpaths or bridleways (of which, more later). Hikers pretend to follow these. Those following grey dotted or dashed lines are usually found following borough or county council boundaries.

Blue lines Either motorways or rivers. One of the better ways of distinguishing between the two is to look out for service stations. Most rivers don't have service stations.

Red triangles Both 'red' and 'triangle' usually mean danger. On a map it means 'Youth Hostel'. Avoid these at all costs unless you want to be asphyxiated by the aroma emanating from 89 pairs of socks belonging to teenagers who failed to convince their parents that the Duke of Edinburgh's Award scheme was not their idea of fun.

FB (Footbridge) A bit like rural buses – there's never one around when you need it. Always check your map to see if your path crosses a blue wavy line. If there isn't an 'FB' marked next to it, take a detour, unless you enjoy swimming.

Cross on a square box A church with a tower.

Cross on a blob A church with a spire. Bluffers passing a church with a spire and expecting to see a church with a tower should call in and pray for alternative directions.

PC (Public Conveniences) These are for wimps. Real hikers go behind a bush.

Brown wavy lines Contour lines that link together points of land at the same height. This is actually vital information. Hikers may become temporarily misplaced from time to time, but they always know whether they should be going up- or downhill. Experienced bluffers will appreciate that one of the joys of going uphill is that there will come a point when it will be necessary to go back down. On many topographic maps, the difference in height between two brown wavy lines is 5m (16ft). However, in practice, there is only one vital piece of information that you need to remember about contour lines: the closer the lines are to each other, the steeper the climb or descent.

Blue wavy lines Seasoned hikers look for the little blue wavy lines in mountainous areas denoting streams. A method to find out (by merely looking at the map) which way the stream is flowing is to notice that when a contour line crosses a blue wavy line it forms a V, and this V always points upstream.

Bluffers will also remember from school science lessons that gravity ensures water runs downhill. Therefore, if a blue wavy line gets thicker, you should be able to work out which way is downstream. This is even easier if you happen to be standing in a stream at the time. Bluffers should never be seen throwing a 'Pooh stick' into the water to determine which way a stream flows.

SCALES

It is important that you should understand your scales. However, this has nothing to do with singing 'The Happy Wanderer' while traipsing gaily through the hills. It's the relationship between the distance on the ground and the distance on the map.

For a map to be of use to a hiker, the distances between two points on it need to be accurate. If a hiker wants to walk from point A to point B, he or she should be able to calculate the distance on the map, and then calculate what the real distance is on the ground. So if the map has a scale of one inch to one mile, and the distance between two points on a map is one inch, it means that the distance on the ground is one mile.

Theoretically.

But because one rarely walks in a straight line, it will usually be a good deal further (especially if one becomes temporarily misplaced before reaching point B).

Always remember, though, if asked how far there is to go, you shouldn't give a distance in miles. Instead, hold your hand up, create a gap between your thumb and index finger, breathe in through gritted teeth before saying, 'According to the map, about that far.'

NAISMITH'S RULE

If you're huddled round a roaring log fire, sampling the local brew in a quiet hikers' pub, and you drop the phrase 'Naismith's Rule' into the conversation, you will instantly command the attention of any hiking aficionados who happen to be listening. But before you do, it's best to understand what it is you're talking about.

In its simplest form, the problem with maps is that they are two-dimensional. Lay them on a table and the only ridges to be seen are the creases where they fold. Contour lines may show peaks and valleys, but when you measure the distance from A to B all you have is the distance on a flat surface. No hike is as flat as a pub tabletop (with a couple of beer mats under the wobbly leg).

Guessing how long it will take you to travel the distance isn't easy. A three-mile walk along a Norfolk lane may only take you an hour. A three-mile climb up a 2,500-foot Scottish hillside will probably take a lot longer than that, particularly if the contour lines are ominously close together.

Ergo this chap, William Naismith, came up with his own proposal, suggesting that:

a) You should allow one hour for every three miles measured on the map.

b) You should add an extra half-hour for every 1,000 feet climbed.

So by Naismith's Rule, the three-mile, 2,500-foot climb would take one hour and 15 minutes longer to complete than the three-mile Norfolk lane walk. Quietly mentioning that Naismith knew all about Scottish inclines because he was one of the 1889 founders of the Scottish Mountaineering Club will further establish your credentials.

TRANTER'S VARIATIONS

Scotsman Phillip Tranter made the realisation that Naismith's timings assumed that everyone had the same fitness level, whereas any bluffer knows that some people can carry eight pints on a tray, while others can only manage three.

Tranter's Variations is a complicated formula enabling hikers to assess their own level of fitness – something with which you need not concern yourself. It gets complicated because it also factors into the equation the weight of the rucksack a hiker is carrying, the weather conditions and the ground conditions underfoot. The knowledge that this variation exists is sufficient to bluff other hikers into thinking that you know your stuff.

Dropping Tranter into any conversation practically guarantees you a pint in the next round of drinks.

NATIONAL GRID

This has nothing to do with walking underneath electricity pylons, but is a system of identifying a specific location on a map to within 100m (328ft). It also provides the 'temporarily misplaced' hiker with the perfect excuse in claiming to suffer from a mild form of dyslexia.

Each map is divided into 1km (0.6-mile) squares by a series of lines running left to right and top to bottom, creating a grid system across the map. Each horizontal and vertical line is numbered between 00 and 99. Always refer to the horizontal lines as 'eastings' and the vertical ones as 'northings'. Those who call them 'horizontals' or 'verticals' will soon find themselves ostracised by hikers in the hope that they will get lost (and they probably will).

Hikers swap grid references like some people swap phone numbers.

Identifying a spot on the map is fairly straightforward. Simply quote the associated numbers of the nearest northing and easting: 4819, for example. However, hikers can be quite fastidious and like to be precise, particularly if there's a 305m (1,000ft) drop in the same grid square. So they subdivide these larger squares with 10 more imaginary vertical and horizontal lines, and use the number from each of these lines to create an extra digit to the easting and the northing. This enables the hiker to give out the preferred 'six-figure grid reference', such as 482198.

Hikers swap grid references like some people swap phone numbers. Getting the two mixed up can be embarrassing, especially if asking whether Lord Hereford's Knob is worth mounting in the Black Mountains.

But that isn't the end of this ramble around the national grid. With an easting and northing line for every kilometre and the requirement to number them with only two digits (00 to 99), these numbers are soon repeated. Once they get to 99, they start numbering again from 00.

Therefore, the six-figure grid reference 482198 is actually repeated several times across the country.

To resolve this problem, each group of 100 eastings and northings is allocated its own two-letter reference. Think of it like an area dialling code. When it's quoted with the six-figure grid reference, hikers can give accurate and unique map references. The right two-letter code should be noted on the map you're using.

What many hikers fail to divulge is that it is very easy to get eastings and northings confused. Inadvertently swapping the two can leave one in a completely different area of the country.

Such confusion is further compounded by an extended pub lunch.

Bluffers who experience a similar difficulty will be pleased to know that there is an easier way to recall the correct method, although you won't find it quoted on a map or muttered in a pub. Hikers would never dream of admitting to the use of memory techniques for their sport.

The perfect grid reference is created by going: *along the corridor* (eastings) and *up the stairs* (northings). Where you go after that is entirely up to you and at your own risk. Bluffers armed with all this knowledge can pick the right map reference with confidence.

ORDNANCE SURVEY MAPS

Britain is blessed with superb maps. Most people are familiar with the Ordnance Survey but may not know how it came into being. You, of course, can enlighten them with the following background information.

When the French were busy storming the Bastille in the late 18th century, the ministers at the Board of Ordnance (the Ministry of Defence) were worried that they would invade and spread revolt in Britain too. It was therefore imperative that England's vulnerable south coast should be accurately mapped in order to prepare the country's defences.

The Board of Ordnance duly carried out the survey and the first Ordnance Survey map was produced in 1801. It covered Kent at a scale of one inch to one mile, and rumours that it included the outline route for sections of the M25 were dispelled when the faint circular marks in the upper left-hand corner of the map closest to London were identified as tea stains from the bottom of carelessly placed cups.

Carrying the War Department's broad arrow heraldic mark as their logo, Ordnance Survey maps come in a variety of scales. Hikers tend to use either the Landranger series or the Explorer series for their treks. That way, should a bluffer meet up with other hikers en route, all will be singing from the same hymn sheet. *Val de ree, val der ra, ha, ha, ha* … (Bluffers should profess at least some familiarity with the lyrics of 'The Happy Wanderer'.)

LANDRANGER

With pretty pink covers, the Landranger series covers the entire British Isles in 204 sheets at a scale of 2cm to 1km (1¼ inches to one mile). However, they tend to be used by indolent hikers who like to leave them lying around to make it look as though they are more active than they actually are.

EXPLORER

This is the more serious hiker's map. Serious because at twice the scale (4cm to 1km/2½ inches to one mile), each sheet generally covers half the area of a Landranger map, but at twice the detail. Clad in fetching psychedelic orange covers, there are 403 sheets to collect – and yes, serious hikers do collect them all. Not only that, they usually keep them filed in numerical order for ease of reference. Hikers who can lay their hands on the right sheet waste less time.

This has little to do with being methodical and more to do with following a logical sequence of steps. Having the right map in the first place dramatically reduces the risk of being temporarily misplaced.

ACTIVE

This is more serious than the serious hiker's Explorer map. An Active map is an existing Landranger or Explorer sheet that has been covered in plastic, making it waterproof and more durable. Meet a hiker using one of these maps, and you should doff your walking hat in respect. For in the rear window of their car, back at the car park, will probably be a sticker declaring 'Active map hikers do it in all weathers!' Bluffers should arm themselves with one immediately.

HARVEY MAPS

Established in 1977, these maps are compiled by hikers themselves, and leave out much of the detail found on

Ordnance Survey maps that hikers find of no interest, such as administrative boundaries, tourist information and the nearest Little Chef. Instead of covering the whole of Britain, as the Ordnance Survey does, Harvey maps concentrate on popular walking areas like Scotland, the Lake District, the Brecon Beacons, and other national parks and long-distance footpaths.

However, intelligent novices will by now have learned an important tip in the art of bluffing. Harvey maps are found in dedicated hiking shops and are produced by hikers for hikers, so should you find yourself in an area covered by a Harvey map, you will immediately gain respect from other hikers if it's a Harvey that you whip out of your rucksack. It has even more bluffing value than an Active map.

STRAIGHT LINE HIKING

Such is a hiker's love of maps that their close scrutiny (of the map, not the hiker – never closely scrutinise a hiker) often leads to the country's official mapmaker being asked some bizarre questions, including *'What is the longest distance you can walk in a straight line in the UK without crossing a road?'*

Whether any hiker is capable of walking in a straight line, particularly having already stopped off at the last three pubs, is up for debate. However, this is just the sort of question that may arise during a pub quiz while you happen to be deservedly quenching your thirst. So, for those bluffers keen to impress their fellow team members, and everyone else at the bar, the distance to remember is 71.5km.

The problem with such questions is that the answer in itself is never enough. So before anyone has a chance to ask a supplementary question, hit them with the following facts.

That the 71.5km straight-line route crosses some of the wildest landscape in Scotland's Cairngorm National Park. Starting from the A9 near the Pass of Drumochter, the route ploughs through the Cairngorms and Grampian mountains. Maintaining a perfect straight line also involves wading several rivers before it finishes just where the Delavine Burn meets an old military road by the River Don near the village of Corgaff. (The beauty of this is that your audience will assume you've walked this route. Mention that the Delavine Burn actually fords the military road (as close scrutiny of the map will reveal). You can even exaggerate how deep that ford is, if you like, because Google Streetview hasn't bothered mapping this particular military road, so it's not easy for your audience to double check.

The cunning bluffer will now realise that because this answer pertains only to Scotland, if an Englishman and a Welshman happen to be in the same pub they will undoubtedly want to know the longest straight-line routes in their home nations.

Fear not, for you can satisfy their thirst for such knowledge with 29.87km and 22.24km respectively. England's straight wander lies in Cumbria and leaves the B6276 near Hazel Bank, north of Brough, and cuts across Warcop Fell, Dufton Fell and the Pennine Way to join the A686 near Leadgate.

The Welsh route begins on a minor lane approximately

three miles north of Beulah and heads no.
towards a minor road near Ffair-Rhos, passing close
the Claerwen Reservoir. This provides a useful clue that
the route involves walking across some of the wettest
mountainous areas of mid-Wales.

You can afford to be vague about the precise
routes for, unlike Scotland with its right to roam,
these English and Welsh options might involve the
occasional crossing of private land, and trespassing is
never acceptable behaviour from a true hiker. Unless
it is absolutely necessary. One should always respect
a private landowner, particularly those wielding
shotguns. If you should encounter one who appears to
be particularly irate, pretend to be Canadian. Everybody
likes Canadians, and they tend to know more about
the Great Outdoors than any other nation. Stick to
superlatives about the beauty of the landscape, heartfelt
apologies about your unfamiliarity with the topography,
and something complimentary and flattering along
the lines of 'Sir/Madam, first may I congratulate you
for your mighty fine work in protecting this mighty
fine part of the world; and second might I apologise on
behalf of my friends and I for any inconvenience we
might have caused you.' It'll also do no harm to dab
your eyes and confide that your grandfather visited the
area just before he took part in the D-Day landings, and
that you promised to pay his respects … and so on. With
luck you'll be offered a lift in the Land Rover back to the
homestead, and a free lunch.

Bear in mind that this ruse is unlikely to work on
some nice gentlemen in camouflage clothing carrying

Glock 17 semi-automatic pistols as you approach the Ministry of Defence's Training Grounds near Warcop.

Straight-line walking may be quickest, but it isn't necessarily the safest.

COMPASSES

You are not going to impress anyone by saying that the sun rises in the east and sets in the west. You're expected to know this. And knowing your north-north-west from your west-south-west sounds knowledgeable but may have other walking-boot enthusiasts thinking you have a nautical or meteorological bent – although forecasting a potential storm coming up from the south-south-west will be met with some admiration if this happens to be true.

Hikers tend to navigate in degrees (of accuracy), rather than compass points. There is one vital piece of information you need to remember at all times. If you have a compass and don't know how to use it, NEVER try to bluff your way out of a situation when you are temporarily misplaced and in thick cloud or fog. To navigate using this equipment and a map, when blind to your surroundings, is a skilled art that takes practice.

Should you anticipate such a situation, try to ensure that you are with other hikers. Then you can explain that your compass 'appears to be faulty with extra air bubbles in the housing'. This enables you to pass the responsibility on to someone else while suggesting that you're also thinking of other hikers' safety. No hiker would use faulty equipment to lure others into danger, even if you don't much care for their company.

Hikers who know how to use a compass will take a bearing. This is the difference between north and the direction of your target destination. For example, if you want to aim for a pub that is directly east, the direction you need to travel is 90° from the direction of north. This means that if you hold your compass in front of you, keep the needle pointing north, and walk at an angle of 90° to the needle, you should reach your destination pub.

This is why hikers go on long pub crawls. The constant sampling of real ale (a hiker wouldn't dream of drinking anything out of a can, or anything that smacks of 'lager'), can interfere with a hiker's ability to hold a compass steady. This could result in becoming temporarily misplaced. The problem with bearings is that a very minor mistake can lead to a major disaster. A bearing that is 2° out sounds minimal, particularly when you remember that there are 360° in a full circle. However, the further the distance travelled, the greater the error. On a long hike an entire pub may be missed. God forbid.

If you started at point A and were aiming for point B but your bearing was 2° out, you would end up at point C. Over a distance of 10km (6 miles), point C is 350m (1,148ft) away from point B. This doesn't sound like much, but if you use the hiking technique of 'upscaling' to make the distance sound further than it really is, you could claim that it is 'more than a third of a kilometre away'.

Notice that as well as quoting the distance in the next unit of measurement, 'upscaling' requires adding phrases of generalisation, such as 'more than'.

With a 2° error, in a best-case scenario you could

end up in the wrong pub. In a worst-case scenario, you might have dropped over a cliff edge to your death.

In this situation, bluffing becomes more difficult.

North, north and north

Never cry, 'Which way is north?' because hikers will realise that you are not really 'one of them'. When you want to know which way north is, you must make it clear to which north you are referring. Why have one, when you could have three?

Magnetic north

This is the north that the little red needle in your compass will point to. Unfortunately, magnetic north doesn't stay still. The magnetic north pole was first discovered in 1831. When explorers went back in 1904 they found that it had moved by more than 48km (30 miles). Recent studies have shown that over the last 150 years, magnetic north has shifted more than 1,088km (680 miles) to the east. And now, magnetic north's speed of eastward travel has increased by nearly 64km (40 miles) a year, forcing some geophysicists to believe the Earth's magnetic fields are about to flip.

This 'polar reversal' will present you with an invaluable opportunity to underline your bluffing credentials by pointing out knowledgeably that magnetic north has swapped places with its opposing south many times during the planet's existence – although the last such reversal happened some 780,000 years ago. And you might add that compass needles have never pointed to that frozen North Pole sitting on the top of the world.

Grid north
This refers to the grid lines running top to bottom down a map, used as the northings for any map references.

True north
The North Pole, which is of no use to hikers whatsoever, except for those doing a polar hike.

The differences between all three varieties of north are usually indicated on the map that hikers use, but as we've seen, the variation of magnetic north is constantly changing, so the variation mentioned on a map is likely to be inaccurate.

Hikers can resolve this by searching for the Pole Star, but this is only of use if you get lost at night. The Pole Star sits directly above the earth's North Pole, give or take a couple of degrees.

In light of all these variations, it really is somewhat surprising that hikers actually manage to arrive at any of their destinations. Of course, it enables you to add one more line of defence when temporarily misplaced:

'Magnetic north isn't in the same place it was the last time I was here!'

You will realise that telling an angry landowner that the sign really should read 'Trespassers will be sued', not 'Trespassers will be prosecuted', is ill-advised, especially if he is pointing a shotgun at you.

THE ONE TRUE WAY

The more astute bluffer will be aware that a footpath does not have to exist on the ground for it to be a legal right of way. This is why maps show footpaths crossing rivers when there is no bridge. Just because there is a right of way doesn't mean that you can physically exercise your right.

All land is owned by someone, whether it is a private individual, a company, a local authority, a charitable organisation or, in the UK, the Crown (which owns quite a lot). Footpaths that are legal rights of way give anyone the right to cross that land on that path without fear of trespassing, as long as they don't wander off the path.

Trespassing is usually a civil matter, not a criminal offence. If you do trespass, you could be sued for damages in the civil courts rather than be prosecuted in the criminal courts. Warning signs saying 'Trespassers will be prosecuted' are therefore technically inaccurate, although such signs tend to be installed by landowners who don't appreciate forthright conversations with hikers who point out the finer aspects of the law. You will realise that telling an angry landowner that the sign really should read 'Trespassers will be sued' is ill-advised, especially if he is pointing a shotgun at you.

Of course, there are exceptions to every rule, and trespassing can be a criminal offence if you're caught wandering along railways or through military training areas. Wisdom would suggest that it is not in a bluffer's interest to be trespassing in such areas anyway, particularly if you're interested in self-preservation.

IN ENGLAND AND WALES

While on a right of way, you, as a hiker, are entitled to:
* pass along the path
* re-pass along the path – in other words you can walk in either direction an unlimited number of times (although this is most likely to happen if you are temporarily misplaced)
* stop to admire the view and take photographs
* stop to have a bite to eat or drink – but you may not cause a blockage (this refers to you physically blocking the right of way, as opposed to the effects of the low fibre content of your packed lunch)
* use any 'natural accompaniment' – for example, items such as pushchairs and wheelchairs ... even a dog. However, being entitled to take a pushchair doesn't mean there is any certainty that you will be able to get it down the path. And being entitled to take a dog doesn't mean it will loyally accompany you. It might have more sense.

Definitive maps

First off, definitive maps aren't definitive. This has nothing to do with the fact that they are maintained by local authorities. It was an attempt by the government in 1949 to clarify the law of paths and rights of way that created these ambiguous 'definitive' maps. County councils were given the legal responsibility of administering a map, detailing all the rights of way in their area. The only way to do this was to consult the local parishes and communities, and then try to identify a compromise where disputes arose. As a result, some rights of way were mistakenly omitted while others that weren't rights of way in the first place were included.

This means that if a path appears on a definitive map, it's evidence of a legal right of way, even if it wasn't such before said map was drawn up. However, if a right of way doesn't appear on a definitive map, this doesn't mean it definitely isn't a right of way; it might be. But then again, it might not be. It's also possible for new rights of way to be created, and these won't show on definitive maps until someone gets around to updating them. The bluffer will note that the dictionary definition of 'definitive' has broadened (even though the paths haven't).

If members of the public have used a path for 20 years without being challenged, thinking that it is a right of way, the law assumes that the landowner intended the path to be used in this way, even if it has not been declared a right of way. So next time the postman hops over your garden fence as a shortcut to deliver your neighbour's post, consider how long he has been doing this before setting your dog loose on him.

Non-hikers tend to think that a footpath is a footpath. That's like saying a country lane is the same as a motorway, simply because it is possible to drive a car down both of them.

A right of way can be designated as any of the following:

* a footpath
* a bridleway
* a RUPP (this has since been renamed a restricted byway)
* a BOAT
* a permissive path.

These varieties in footpath classification are recorded on maps, and therefore supposedly assist hikers with navigation. Experienced hikers (and knowledgeable bluffers) tend to reclassify them as one of the following:

* overgrown
* passable
* a country lane that the highways department has forgotten and which is now blocked by an HGV driver who believed the sat nav on his dashboard was correct
* routes requiring an 'every man for himself' approach
* a nice idea in principle.

Footpaths
These do exactly what they say on the tin. They are paths for feet. Only people (and any natural accompaniment) may use them.

Bridleways

A bridleway is a bonus for hikers because walkers can use them as well as cyclists and horse riders. However, even a detailed map won't tell you about the cross-country biker just about to hit you as he comes around the next corner.

RUPPs

The acronym for Road Used as a Public Path. Technically, it is a road, and therefore motorised vehicles are permitted, although they are generally so poorly maintained that no sensible driver would consider taking a vehicle down them; the puddle-filled potholes would very effectively succeed in shafting your big end.

In practice, such routes tend only to be used by hikers, cyclists and horse riders, and since the Countryside and Rights of Way (CRoW) Act 2000, all remaining RUPPs were reclassified as restricted byways on 2 May 2006. A bluffer will boost his or her status by knowing what they are when they are spotted on signposts and waymarks (*see* 'Close Encounters of the Herd Kind', page 101), and will insist on referring to them by their former name.

BOATs

BOATs are not the sections of footpaths that cross water. They are Byways Open to All Traffic, more simply referred to as 'byways'. In other words, it's every hiker for himself. Not only may you meet other walkers but also cyclists, horse riders and motorised vehicles that still have their big ends intact. Like RUPPs, BOATs tend not to be maintained to a high-enough standard for ordinary vehicles to use them for the weekly shopping trip. On the other hand, drivers of 4 x 4s love them. Never argue with a 'Chelsea tractor' on a BOAT, particularly one with bull bars. The drivers generally have no idea what they're doing.

Permissive paths

There's a fine line between permissiveness and flirtation, and a permissive path may cross this line on a regular basis. Such paths are not legal rights of way; they merely tease the hiker into thinking they are. One day you can walk along one, the next day it may be closed. One minute it's your best pal, the next it just doesn't want to know you.

Bluffers are encouraged to embrace the permissive path. You never know what joys and personal pleasures it may bring. Permissive paths (and bridleways) are offered by liberal-minded landowners who want to share their land with others. However, behind every enlightened landowner is a narrow-minded solicitor, determined not to let his client's generosity be turned against him. It's the legal beagle's advice to close the permissive path for at least one day a year to prevent the 20-year rule from applying – which means you can't use it on the only day of the year you really need to.

Open access

Many hikers have been crowing about the CRoW Act 2000 because of the freedom it gives to wander freely across areas of:

* mountain
* moorland
* heathland
* downland
* registered common land
* crumbling clifftop.

Commonly referred to as the 'right to roam', it means that in England and Wales there are now a further 3.4 million acres in which to get lost (sorry, temporarily misplaced). Bluffers will be aware that it is not a right to roam at will across these newly designated areas. It actually offers managed and controlled access on foot.

Just like permissive paths, open-access land can be closed by the landowner for up to 28 days a year, or longer for certain safety or conservation reasons. Joyfully, though, this right of access is only for hikers. Horse riders and cyclists can only cross such land if a bridleway, restricted byway or BOAT crosses the area. If it does, they can't deviate from it. Hikers, on the other hand, can walk across such land safe in the knowledge that they won't get mown down by a 4 x 4. Unless, of course, the landowner drives one (and normally does).

The Kinder Trespass
Shrewd bluffers will have gathered by now that there is periodic friction between hikers and landowners. Hikers are not normally a militant bunch, but the open-access land enjoyed today may not have come about if it hadn't been for a bunch of hard-core hikers out for a walk on 24 April 1932. That's when 400 of them set off

from Bowden Bridge quarry to climb to the summit of Kinder Scout, the highest point in Derbyshire. Working on the principle of safety in numbers, they survived an altercation with the Duke of Devonshire's gamekeepers halfway up their ascent (although one of the gamekeepers claimed to suffer a slight injury) and continued to meet up on the summit with some hikers from Sheffield who'd trespassed from nearby Edale. When they returned to civilisation, five of them were arrested and subsequently charged on the grounds of unlawful assembly and breach of the peace. They were imprisoned for between two and six months.

You shouldn't be fooled into thinking that 'open-access land' is always open, or accessible.

This outraged the public, and the campaign for a right to roam gained momentum. A few weeks later, 10,000 hikers assembled for another rally in Winnats Pass, near Castleton, Derbyshire. You should make a mental note never to annoy a dyed-in-the-wool hiker. While they may appear to be a solitary wanderer, their camaraderie means they can raise more troops than a small African nation.

The government, having been distracted by the Second World War, realised that something had to be done. So it created the 'definitive map' disaster and passed legislation creating the national parks – but nothing was said about the right to roam. It was only in 2000 that legislation was passed that allowed hikers to reach their roaming destination. Government officials were presumably 'temporarily misplaced' on a regular basis while implementing the law, seeing as the right didn't come into effect until 2005.

You shouldn't be fooled into thinking that 'open-access land' is always open, or accessible. In fact, any 'open-access land' designated on your map with a Ready Brek orange glow around its perimeter may include the following, all of which are out of bounds to hikers:

* buildings
* land that is within 20m (65ft) of a building containing livestock, or a house
* land beneath electricity pylons or wind turbines
* quarries
* golf courses/racecourses
* aerodromes
* arable land
* a couple of muddy fields in Somerset during the Glastonbury Festival.

Look for the white disc with a brown hiker walking on brown hills, created to advise hikers when they are entering open-access land. When you leave such land you may spot a similar sign with a red diagonal line across it to denote the fact that open-access freedom no longer applies. Alternatively, there may be a landowner-improvised sign telling you, in the politest possible terms, to go away.

IN SCOTLAND

North of Hadrian's Wall, Scottish hikers have been wandering aimlessly for years, thanks to their more relaxed trespass laws. Here, landowners can only sue trespassers for actual damage caused, or if the trespasser is caught chasing game (e.g., animals or birds). Because of this, hikers had unhindered access until the arrival of the Land Reform (Scotland) Act 2003, which clarified responsibilities for both landowners and anyone accessing the countryside. At 74 pages long, it has been very helpful to hikers. The number of trees felled to produce the paper to print it on has helped open up more views across the country.

For a right of way to exist in Scotland, it must have been used for at least 20 years and link two public places, which presumably includes public houses (useful for hikers who don't like coming to an abrupt halt in the middle of a cornfield). Scottish rights of way are classified as:

* vindicated (where a court has confirmed that it is a right of way)
* asserted (where landowners accept that the path is a right of way, and saved themselves the expense of going to court to get it vindicated)
* claimed (where a right of way meets other Scottish common-law requirements of a right of way, but a court hasn't vindicated it, nor has the landowner asserted it).

All this vindication, assertiveness and propensity to claim suggests a certain amount of bloody-mindedness among Scottish hikers. But don't worry: it's just the way they speak. It's estimated that only 1% of Scottish rights of way are vindicated, and 15% have been asserted, so mathematically skilled bluffers will immediately spot that the remaining 84% are only claiming to be rights of way. Therefore, statistically, a Scottish hiker is more likely to sight a Scottish golden eagle than find a vindicated Scottish right of way.

Tackling a long-distance route gives you hours of pleasure for months beforehand as you plan your route in meticulous detail in the pub over a pint or three.

GOING THE DISTANCE

Not all hikers enjoy roaming about for a mere few hours. Some like hiking for more than one day in a row. They aren't masochists (well, not all of them). You might wonder why anyone would want to get up and start walking when their feet still ache from the 32km (20 miles) they trekked yesterday. But tackling a long-distance route is popular with many hikers because it gives you:

* a sense of achievement upon completion
* sights that aren't possible from a bus or car
* hours of pleasure for months beforehand as you plan your route in meticulous detail in the pub over a pint or three (depending on how much detail you want to go into)
* an opportunity to travel in the way your ice age ancestors did (without having to slay any woolly mammoths en route)
* blisters on your blisters, located on bits of one's body that were previously unknown or unappreciated.

At the last count, there were more than 1,300 long-distance hiking routes criss-crossing the UK, ranging from under 16km (10 miles) to over 1,600km (1,000 miles). Should the uninitiated enquire how this can be when Land's End to John o'Groats is only about 1,300km (850 miles), you will point out that the length of the British coastline is 17,819.88km (11,072.76 miles) – and that's just the island of Great Britain, so it doesn't include the other estimated 6,209 islands.

You might also point out with modest authority that you can't be absolutely sure of the accuracy of the decimal point, because coastal erosion might have altered it since you last checked. It's this sort of attention to detail that will enable you to boost your standing among fellow hikers beyond measure.

On the other hand, serious hikers will tell you that everything is measurable.

NATIONAL TRAILS

The crème de la crème of long-distance routes are the National Trails. These are the most famous names, the ones that are funded by central government. Think of them as the motorways of the hiking world. In fact, some are so popular that sections of the busiest routes are almost as wide as a motorway due to the impact of all those hiking boots.

You should note that some trails are more challenging than others and are scored accordingly, allowing you to be properly prepared should you find yourself in conversation with a National Trail techie. For the purposes of our National Trail Scale, assume that 10 is a route likely to be any hardened hiker's Achilles heel, while a zero is something they're more likely to consider attempting in flip-flops.

South West Coast Path

The South West Coast Path stretches 1,015km (630 miles) from Minehead in Somerset, around Land's End and finishes at Poole Harbour in Dorset. It used to be just over 805km (500 miles) in length, but that aforementioned coastal erosion means that the path keeps getting diverted, which is why it has grown.

Tackle this, and not only will you have walked 1,015km, but you will have ascended umpteen cliffs. The total height climbed is over 35,000m (114,830ft). Everest is 8,848m (29,029ft) high, so it might be easier to think of the South West Coast Path as the equivalent of climbing just under four Everests. Most hikers love this sort of analogy.

Rating A 10 on our National Trail Scale, but probably a 15 in reality.

Pennine Way

This was the first, and is probably the most famous, National Trail. At 430km (268 miles) long, it follows the backbone of Britain while making some serious demands on your own.

Rating A good 8 or 9, but do claim it as a 10 if tackled in winter.

Pembrokeshire Coast Path

This scenic path follows the beautiful Pembrokeshire

coast for 300km (186 miles). Just close your eyes when passing the oil refineries of Milford Haven.

Rating Coastal trails mean cliff climbs and death-defying cliff drops. It's an 8.

Thames Path

The Thames Path is a more sedate 296km (184 miles) from the Thames Barrier to the source of this great river near Lechlade in the Cotswolds. It allows hikers to recreate *Three Men in a Boat*, without getting as wet.

Rating It's a 1, but only because of a particularly nasty muddy patch just north of Oxford.

Offa's Dyke Path

When it comes to building barriers that separate countries, Offa, king of Mercia in the late 8th century, could have taught Hadrian a thing or two about keeping out annoying neighbours. Offa's Dyke may be made of earth but the trail still rambles for 285km (177 miles) along most of the England–Wales border, which is over twice as long as Hadrian's efforts.

Rating A sweat-inducing 8, because the Welsh Borders are more challenging than many think.

Glyndwr's Way

Glyndwr's Way takes a circuitous route from Knighton and travels for 217km (135 miles) around mid-Wales to finish at Welshpool, less than 48km (30 miles) further north along the England–Wales border. It's called 'going the pretty way'.

Rating A 7, although it has sections that are worthy of a 9, particularly if you happen to bump into enthusiasts re-enacting Glyndwr and his Welsh soldiers, and you happen to be English.

Cleveland Way

At 175km (109 miles) in length, the Cleveland Way skirts around the North York Moors, thus avoiding all those day-tripping cars on the A170 to Scarborough.

Rating A picturesque 6, with plenty of opportunities to stop for fish and chips along the coastal section.

Cotswold Way

This follows the escarpment of the Cotswold hills for most of its 164km (102-mile) length. Appropriately, the trail ends in Bath, where you can enjoy a soothing, long, hot soak.

Rating A surprising 7, because the route encounters Cooper's Hill, the site of the annual Cheese-rolling Championships, used because of its one-in-one gradient (45° angle).

North Downs Way

Runs 246km (153 miles) from Farnham to Dover. Such is its proximity to civilisation that hikers are less than 90 minutes from a Pret A Manger at any point en route.

Rating A 4, on the grounds that you can't really rate it as a gruelling 'off the beaten track' hike.

South Downs Way

An opportunity to share 160 km (100 miles) with hordes of cyclists and horse riders. If your legs are playing up, the chances of cadging a lift are good on this route –

if you don't mind riding side-saddle or sitting on the crossbar. The coastal towns of Worthing, Brighton and Eastbourne are all within tantalising sight of the route, and many hikers fall victim to the temptation to visit them for a spot of R&R. Those who do rarely make it back to the top to continue down the way.

Rating A 6, but only if you stay on high ground and don't divert to the seaside.

Peddars Way and Norfolk Coast Path

This East Anglian trail actually starts in Suffolk, heads straight for the coast at Hunstanton and then turns right to Cromer. It's 150 km (93 miles) long and one of its greatest selling points is that it's … flat.

Rating This is a scenically rewarding, physically undemanding 0. Don't forget your flip-flops.

The Ridgeway

Follow in the footsteps of prehistoric man on Britain's oldest road and travel 136km (85 miles) from Overton Hill on the North Wessex Downs to Ivinghoe Beacon on the edge of the Chilterns. Bear in mind, though, that Britain's oldest road is likely to have Britain's oldest potholes. It's a bit hilly in places, but because it's open to cyclists, horse riders and in some places 4 x 4s, the opportunities for hitch-hiking are high.

Rating This is a 4, on the grounds that parts of the road haven't been resurfaced since the Roman Conquest.

Yorkshire Wolds Way

Starts where the Cleveland Way (*see* page 43) leaves

off and cuts across the Yorkshire Wolds for 127km (79 miles) to finish near the Humber Bridge.

Rating A worthy 4, although, at times, when on the tops of the hills 'you can see forever', which can be demoralising when hiking, mainly because of that sinking feeling of not actually getting anywhere.

Hadrian's Wall Path

It's 135km (84 miles) long. Avoid calling 'Halt! Who goes there?' to everyone you meet. It's mildly amusing for the first 3 miles, but by mile 81 your fellow walkers may be fantasising about throwing a well-aimed spear at your back. Despite being 2,000-odd years in the making, they've still only laid the foundations in places.

Rating An invigorating 7.

Wales Coast Path

Earn the admiration of your local pub-quiz team by telling them that in 2012 Wales became the first country in the world to provide a continuous walking route around its entire coastline. Stretching from the Dee Estuary, near Chester, to Chepstow in the Bristol Channel, it is 1,400km (870 miles), so it's not your typical weekend wander.

Rating A perfect 10, although hikers leaving their car at Chester will have to tackle Offa's Dyke to complete the circuit. (Rating for the entire circumnavigation of Wales: 18-plus)

England Coast Path

Exists as a great idea and work is ongoing to create a continuous coastal route, but don't pack your rucksack just yet. A sizeable new section, at Weymouth in Dorset, opened in time for the sailing events of the London 2012 Olympics. Astute bluffers will appreciate the Olympian connection. Completing this new path will be a marathon, not a 4,426km (2,750-mile) sprint. When finished, it will be the longest managed coastal path in the world.

WALKING THE WORLD

It doesn't take a bluffer to acknowledge that British Ordnance Survey maps are the best in the world, or that Britain has the widest variety of hiking landscapes in such a relatively small island. But should you wish to really impress a group of hikers, then draw upon your knowledge of each of the following international hiking trails to demonstrate your walking worldliness.

(And, generally speaking, the golden rule to foreign hiking is that preparation is everything. They don't sell Imodium in Nepal.)

The Inca Trail, Peru – 88.5km (55 miles)

The journey to one of the world's most famous destinations, Machu Picchu, is not for the faint-hearted … or the weak-lunged. Starting at an altitude of 2,600m (8,530ft), it climbs to the highest point of 4,200m (13,779ft) on the second day. That's 1,600m (5,250ft) of climbing. Should you find yourself floundering slightly if questioned by someone who's actually tackled this route, then fall back on the classic altitude sickness excuse that affects so many of the trekkers at this point. It plays havoc with the memory, you will say sadly. The chances of encountering someone who has finished the Inca Trail are increasingly low, for the Peruvian government now limits the number of people permitted to tackle the route in an attempt to cut erosion. Those limits still allow 200 hikers a day to be on the trail, though.

The best time of year to tackle the trail is between March and July, although it's busiest between March and April. If you inadvertently bluff about going in February when the trail is closed to tourists, redeem yourself by explaining that you were part of the official Peruvian government clean-up team who collect the debris left behind by eleven months of hiking tourists.

The Appalachian Trail, USA – 3,525km (2,190 miles)

The Appalachian National Scenic Trail, to give it its full, official name, is one of the world's longest footpaths – although the much-anticipated 4,425km (2,750-mile) England Coastal Path will take this crown when, or if, it is ever completed. Clearly the coastline is already there, but if the same Brexit negotiators are involved with negotiating access rights from existing landowners, then the Appalachian Trail has little to worry about for another century or two. (Note that while some Brexiteers supported a hard cliff-edge Brexit, most hikers would rather not, voluntarily, walk over a cliff edge on any coastal path.)

The trail follows the Appalachian mountains from Springer Mountain in Georgia to Katahdin in Maine.

It attracts over 3 million visitors a year, although it is estimated that only 0.1% of that figure (some 3,000) people actually tackle the whole route in one go. If an Appalachian Trail guru happens to be nearby, tell the rest of your audience that a complete trek along the trail is known as a *thru-hike* and the dedicated trekker is called a *thru-hiker* (among many other names).

Talking of names, thru-hikers are encouraged to create a *trail name* for themselves, instead of using their real name when signing official trail registers along the route. Knowledgable bluffers soon realise that a true hiker selects a name that conveys their love of the great outdoors: *Blisterfeet*, *Trailhugger*, or *Wandering Willy*. Novice hikers, wet behind the ears because they failed to buy the right waterproof headgear, find themselves named by other, passing, hikers en route: *Armpit Rainforest*, *The Dawdler*, or *Chafing Chugger*.

Of course, choosing the right name is one thing, but coming up with a suitable story as to how you acquired that name is another. Not that a bluffer would ever have that problem. (Those who find themselves temporarily and creatively challenged simply need to paste the phrase *Appalachian Trail nickname* into any half-decent web browser.)

Such thru-hikes can take anything between seven months to a year to complete, which is a staggeringly long time for a stroll. (It's a staggeringly long time for staggering, full stop.) To anyone under thirty, a year away from the modern world is more than a lifetime. Time it wrong and you could miss out on the next two launches of the Apple iPhone. And don't even think about all those Windows Updates that will need doing when you return.

As modern equipment goes, the most useful device to have with you on this trail is a whistle. Wild bears don't like noise, so blowing the whistle should warn any bears in the vicinity of your presence, scaring them off. Should you encounter a deaf bear then at least the whistle will help emergency services locate you while you still have enough breath left in your body to blow it.

Bluffers will quickly identify that the safest and far more relaxing way of tackling the trail is to let someone else do it for you ... like Bill Bryson, whose 1998 autobiographical book, *A Walk in the Woods*, recounts his attempt at tackling the trail. (Note the word attempt.)

Those who tackle and survive the whole trail can brag that their total ascent is equivalent to climbing Everest sixteen times.

Everest Base Camp Trek, Nepal – 129km (80 miles)

Of course, climbing the equivalent of Everest so many times is impressive, but not as impressive as going to the real thing. But always remember that a hiker is not a mountaineer, so you wouldn't be expected to strap on your oxygen tanks and scale the highest point on Earth. However, the two-to-three-week return trip from Lukla to Everest Base Camp presents other just as daunting challenges.

While the round-trip trek to Base Camp is roughly 129km (80 miles), it's not the distance that is challenging, but the altitude. If you survive the landing at the infamous Lukla Airport, reputedly the most dangerous airport in the world with its 527m (1,729ft) long runway at a gradient of 11.7%, then all that's left is acclimatising to the starting point altitude of 2,819m (9,250ft) above sea level. Everest Base Camp sits at 5,334m (17,500ft).

It might only be just over 2,515m (8,250ft) of climbing, less than climbing Scotland's Ben Nevis twice, but altitude sickness can kill. On average, between three and five people a year die tackling the Everest Base Camp trek. In bad years it can be as many as 15.

Therefore, the Everest Base Camp trek demands respect. Claim it for your bucket list, but bluffers should remember that it could be the trek where the bucket list claims you.

Kilimanjaro, Northern Tanzania – 64km (40 miles)

There are several routes up Kilimanjaro, so bluffers may wish to tailor their account for different audiences. Like Machu Picchu and Everest, the biggest challenge when trekking to Kilimanjaro's 5,895m (19,341ft) summit is the altitude (again). Longer routes allow more time for hikers to acclimatise to the altitude and, therefore, they have higher success rates.

Hikers tackling the Rongai route have about an 80% success rate of reaching the summit, helped because it takes the drier, northern flank of the mountain.

The Machame route involves crossing the notorious Barranco Wall, a steep section that requires what most hikers would refer to as scrambling, rather than hiking. It is the cheapest route, for it involves camping, rather than hut shelters, which means it's popular with students and other budget hikers.

The Umbwe route is the most technically challenging. Mention this route if sharing a pint with a group of mountaineers, for you will immediately gain their respect. Just mention the exposed ridge on day two known as *Jiwe Kamba*, or Rope Rock, then glance at your hands, as if recalling the lacerations inflicted when you hauled yourself up.

The Shira route begins along a road, and some hikers opt to use 4WD vehicles for this section. This is the bluffers' preferred route. It is also the preferred route of television celebrities and their camera crews (they usually switch off the air con in the vehicles for that hot and sweaty look). The disadvantage of the Shira route is that altitude is gained very quickly, often more quickly than the body can adjust to. But let's face it, a celebrity with altitude sickness usually makes far better television viewing. And viewing is what the bluffer will be doing back in the Shira camp (if you've got any sense).

Overland Track, Tasmania – 64km (40 miles)

This devil of a walk is one of Australia's most famous, crossing many of Tasmania's highest peaks on its journey from Cradle Mountain to Lake St Clair. It's a true wilderness experience for it crosses the Tasmanian Wilderness World Heritage Area, one of the last great expanses of temperate rainforest in the world.

The seasoned bluffer will know that hikers tackling this route between 1 October and 31 May can do so only in a north–south direction. During the summer season hikers must purchase an Overland Pass, which are limited in number.

Talk knowledgeably about the summer snows and recall stoically the broken boardwalk sections that meant wading through ankle-deep mud. Don't forget to produce the toothmarked Bear Grylls Survival Guidebook you used to fight off the notoriously aggressive carnivorous marsupials known as Tasmanian Devils that were trying to steal your food. You might drop casually into conversation that Devils have one of most powerful bite forces of any living mammal, relative to body size. This is because they have heads bigger than a rhino on a body about the size of a Jack Russell. If you choose to pursue this line of bluffing, make sure that you don't fall into the trap of saying that you once wrestled a Tasmanian Tiger to the ground as it tried to make off with a member of your party. Once indigenous to this part of Australia (also a carnivorous marsupial, otherwise known as a thylacine) it has been extinct since 1936.

Should someone mention they're thinking of tackling the OT, nod wisely before leaning closer to them and whispering quietly, 'Salt solution.' Then gravely impart the advice that this is the best way to remove leeches from the skin should they find any such uninvited hitch-hikers. And that's why everyone mentions the broken boardwalks.

Although, as any bluffer knows, that's what all great hikes are about: reconnecting with nature.

The great majority of hikers don't like wind turbines, and so neither must you.

PARK LIFE

Following the kerfuffle in Derbyshire over the Kinder Trespass, the 1949 National Parks and Access to the Countryside Act created a handful of national parks designed to give hikers, and other outdoor enthusiasts, an opportunity to explore some of the best areas the UK has to offer. These national parks are not owned by the state, but by private individuals, businesses and charitable organisations, such as the National Trust. So, when in a national park, a bluffer still needs to know his byways from his permissive paths.

The act saw the creation of national park authorities, whose responsibility it is to protect the natural beauty of the landscape while also promoting the area as an outdoor playground (although any bluffers looking for a quick snog behind the bike sheds may have to use a stone wall instead).

You should be aware that not everyone is happy about the role of national park authorities, because they are also the local planning authority. Locals seeking planning permission for their satellite dish, so they can obtain terrestrial TV signals via traditional transmitters that the mountains often deny them, are understandably upset when their application is rejected on the grounds that they damage the scenic quality of the landscape, yet permission is granted to the local power company to erect 300 wind turbines. (Note that the great majority of hikers don't like wind turbines, and so neither must you.) There are currently 15 national parks in England, Wales and Scotland:

Brecon Beacons
Avoid Sennybridge, an MOD training camp, where any temporarily misplaced hikers can find themselves being shot for having poor navigational skills.

Norfolk Broads
Preferred by hikers with a canoe, instead of walking boots, on each foot.

Cairngorms
A big place, it has Britain's highest and biggest mountain range, and is home to the UK's highest funicular railway.

Dartmoor
Encounter a hiker wearing outdoor clothing with arrows all over it and rejoice, for you've spotted a rare sight: an escaped convict from Dartmoor Prison. Probably wise to hand over your own clothing if requested to do so.

Exmoor
Designated as Europe's first International Dark Sky Reserve, it's the perfect place to hone your Pole Star

navigation skills – assuming it isn't raining when it's dark.

Lake District
Sixteen million visitors a year can't be wrong … at least not about the traffic congestion on the Windermere to Grasmere road.

Loch Lomond and the Trossachs
Whether you take the high road or the low road, never ask a passing hiker if they've lost their trossachs.

New Forest
Created around 1079 by William I as a royal hunting ground, it's about time they dropped the 'new', although it was only designated as a national park in 2005. So in national park terms it's still relatively new.

Northumberland
Sandwiched between the Scottish Borders and Hadrian's Wall, hikers should keep checking over their shoulder in case they find themselves caught in the middle of the next cross-border skirmish.

North Yorkshire Moors
The park where you literally step back in time, especially if crossing the North Yorkshire Moors Railway line with its steam trains, and then drop into Goathland, also known as Aidensfield to fans of a certain 1950s TV drama. (There's no need to switch to 1950s walking clothing, though.)

Peak District

One of the first national parks to be designated as such in 1951, this one comes in two colours: dark and white. The northern (dark) peak is muddy and peaty, whereas the southern (white) peak is rocky. Just like chocolate, there are those who prefer the dark to white, and vice versa. Unlike chocolates, neither has a particularly soft centre.

Pembrokeshire Coast

Britain's only truly coastal national park. The designated park area follows the coastline, so bluffers who casually drop into conversation that its widest point is 16km (10 miles) and its narrowest a mere 100m (328ft) will be held in high esteem by their audience.

Snowdonia

The big brother of Welsh national parks, Snowdonia is home to the tallest mountain in England and Wales (Snowdon), and Wales' largest natural lake (Llyn Tegid). Real hikers always avoid taking the train to the summit of Snowdon, and instead speak of the 'Snowdon Horseshoe', a seven-hour ordeal to be avoided by those afraid of heights.

South Downs

The latest national park baby, born on 1 April 2011, it gives Londoners a national park they can get to in a day – assuming the M25 isn't gridlocked for more than five hours, of course.

Yorkshire Dales

Sandwiched between the Lake District National Park and the North York Moors National Park, it's either a stone-waller's heaven, or hell. The park has 8.5 times more stone walls than hedgerows, and nearly six times more stone walls than footpaths.

AONBs

AONB is not an item on the local parish council agenda, (Any Other Needless Business), but another countryside designation. Lesser-known than the much more famous national parks, an Area of Outstanding Natural Beauty is still a fantastic place to explore on foot, and hikers in the know often choose these over the ever-popular national parks.

Created by the same act that led to national parks, there are 47 AONBs in England, Wales and Northern Ireland. Scenically, they are just as beautiful as their national park cousins; they just don't get the same number of visitors. This is because, while a national park authority has to preserve the landscape and promote the area as an outdoor playground, AONBs are designed to preserve the natural beauty of the area.

Should a hiker mention an AONB they enjoy visiting, a bluffer should always tap the side of their nose, and nod their head to acknowledge that a precious secret has been shared. AONBs are where the *real* hikers go. National parks are for tourists looking for nice views from the car park.

When your granny told you to put a jumper on because you were cold and she was too mean to put another lump of coal on the fire, she was actually training you to be a hiker.

GEAR UP AND GO

THE OUTDOOR GEAR SHOP

Welcome to the place where even dedicated hikers find themselves bluffing at times. Outdoor gear shop assistants fall into two categories: those who thought they were applying for a Saturday job at a bird-food shop (Millets), and those who live, breathe and eulogise about everything to do with the outdoors. It is the latter that the bluffer should be wary of. The former don't last long and quickly move on to the nearest pizza-delivery business, realising that in order for them to survive in the great outdoors, they need a crash helmet and a 50cc bike.

Outdoor gear shop assistants are a fearsome bunch. They are not just healthily fit, they are embarrassingly fit. They all act as if they've done the Three Peaks Challenge – that's Snowdon, Scafell Pike and Ben Nevis – before clocking on for duty.

You can always spot one of this fraternity, especially if you're in an outlet located in the 'outdoorsy' regions of the Lake District, Wales or Scotland, because:

* They are always kitted out in walking boots, even if the entire shop is on the ground floor.
* They wear T-shirts and shorts, even in winter, despite the front doors of the shop being wide open to the elements.
* The T-shirts have 'Hikers do it with their boots on' written across their chest, and 'I'm in front of you – slowcoach' across the back.
* If they need to open a piece of packaging they'll ignore the scissors on the cash desk, and slice it open with one of the Swiss Army knives they have chained to their belt.
* Trainees are easier to spot because they are always roped to a more experienced member of staff for safety reasons. You should know that the recruitment process for most of these employees is unlike that for any other job. Interviews tend to take place at the top of mountains. Bad weather doesn't stop recruitment from taking place. Thick fog merely means that the successful applicant and new boss don't know what the other looks like until they start work, despite having shaken hands and shared hip flasks to seal the deal at the summit.

The typical outdoor gear shop assistant loves his or her job for the following reasons:

* The outdoor clothing for sale in the shop never looks as good on the customer as it does on the assistants – and they know it.

* They know about every item for sale in the shop – they've got one at home (due to the staff discount).
* They enjoy bragging about their latest conquests with their work colleagues (the Pennine Way in two days, Ben Nevis in a force 10 gale), in order to see the looks on customers' faces when they overhear.
* They genuinely enjoy passing on hints, tips and advice to real hikers. Equally, they enjoy winding everybody else up.

This is where you should start bluffing, and on the following pages is all you'll need to know to survive all the way to the cash till.

Stage 1
Start off by mentioning a popular tourist honeypot for hiking and then, in a nonchalant way, drop in a comment that shows how you tackled it out of season, or at a time when most tourists wouldn't even consider doing such a route.

> *'Did Catbells yesterday, early enough to reach the summit and watch the sun rise over Derwent Water. Pure magic.'*

This demonstrates that you're prepared to go that extra mile and are not one of those who wants to look the part even though the longest walk they usually do is from the shop to the car park. Assistants will not hold it against you that you've mentioned a typical touristy place. Everyone has to start somewhere.

Stage 2

Whatever it is you are thinking of buying, suggest that you recently saw a review of it in one of the well-known hiking magazines. Something along the lines of:

> *'I'm looking for a pair of trousers that was reviewed in* Country Walking/Lakeland Walker/TGO (The Great Outdoors) *magazine last month, but I can't remember who they were made by. …'*

This reinforces the message that you're a serious hiker, not a fashion freak who has wandered in off the street. Fashion freaks don't buy these magazines. It also sends an important subliminal message: you can't remember the name of the brand, but you're prepared to listen to the assistant's expert advice.

Stage 3

Give the impression your purchasing decision has been influenced by the shop assistant's advice. Identify the product the assistant thinks is right for you and buy it, while suggesting that you were originally going to buy something different and far cheaper.

> *'So you're saying these trousers, though more expensive, are better than the ones I was originally looking at, because they've got extra protection against UV rays.'*

This will demonstrate that your commitment to hiking is such that extra expense is not really a consideration.

CLOTHING

Gone are the days when you could hike the hills in a tweed jacket and matching trousers, with socks that came up to your armpits. These days, never venture out inappropriately clad unless you know you'll be in thick fog for the duration of your walk, and thus won't be seen.

Learn it now. Cotton, denim and flimsy shoes scream 'City dweller trying to look cool on the hills on a bank holiday Monday.' It's not what your outdoor clothing *says* about you that counts, it's what it *does for you* that matters. Hikers frequently remind themselves quietly, 'There's no such thing as bad weather, only bad clothing choices.' So, to avoid bad choices, bluffers should digest the following topics carefully.

Layers

When your granny told you to put a jumper on because you were cold and she was too mean to put another lump of coal on the fire, she was actually training you to be a hiker. Keeping warm on the hills is all about layers, of which there are four:

1. base
2. mid
3. fleece or soft shell
4. waterproof or outer shell.

The base layer is the most frightening. It hugs your skin – all of it. Rolls of it adhere to your midriff, clinging so as not to get lost.

Hiking can generate half a litre of sweat in an hour. Hike hard across the landscape and this volume of sweat trebles, so technically you're not hiking, but swimming. The base layer shakes off this excess moisture quickly, which is *a good thing* because you don't get that wet, cold clammy feeling when you put your rucksack back on after a break.

If out on the hills without a fleece, don't worry: there are always a few spare sheep wandering around.

Outdoor gear assistants will refer to this as the 'wicking effect': the transfer of moisture from your body to the outside elements. They may turn their noses up at this for two reasons. First, being in the stressful location of an outdoor gear shop may cause your body to 'wick' your own natural aroma around the shop. Second, the assistants don't actually sweat themselves. They are so fit that breaking into a mild perspiration hasn't happened to them since they hiked from John o'Groats to Land's End one wet Wednesday afternoon.

The mid-layer looks more like ordinary clothing. It comes disguised as T-shirts, shirts, blouses, trousers, skirts and shorts in either earthy, natural or vibrant, psychedelic colours. (There's no middle ground in outdoor clothing colours.) Never mention to the shop assistant that you've got a shirt at home that looks 'just like that one on the rails over there'; you haven't. They might all look as if they're made from natural fabrics, but space-age technology has been applied. Even if the shirt in your cupboard was bought from an outdoor gear shop, it's last year's technology, whereas everything on the rails in front of you is this year's.

Depending upon which season is taking place in the great outdoors, the fleece or soft-shell layer may be either the final layer in the system or the penultimate one. Fleece jumpers or coats work just like the fleece on a sheep (but smell better). Dense fibres trap the warmth of your body, preventing it from escaping, and also help to cut out the wind. If out on the hills without a fleece, don't worry: there are always a few spare sheep wandering around. Just catch a couple, strap one across your chest, and another across your back, and you'll enjoy the same benefits. Sheep have a nervous habit of urinating when hikers pass by, so strap them head upwards and feet outwards. There's only so much work your wicking base layer can do.

The waterproof or outer-shell layer is what most non-hikers would call a coat. It's usually a noisy garment that rustles loudly when you swing your arms as you stroll purposefully along the footpath. The outer layer should keep you dry when it is raining/hailing/snowing, and keep you warm in a gale-force wind. Bluffers who are now thinking about the moisture being wicked away from their bodies by the base layer need not worry. You might be hiking through a particularly vicious anticyclone high on the moors, but all these layers should work together to prevent a similar anticyclone from taking up residence beneath your outer layer. Thankfully, the manufacturers have devised a high-tech solution to this problem. It's called a zip.

Actually, manufacturers have pioneered a variety of materials designed to let your clothes breathe out any moisture you create without letting in any of the moisture that nature creates. 'Breathability' is all to do with making the holes that let the moisture out smaller than the rain molecules that want to get in.

Both manufacturers and outdoor gear shops are keen to use buzzwords when describing their products, so the sooner you latch on to these, the better.

Activewear Designed to make you think that your clothes are working harder than you are.

Solar drying When the sun comes out, it'll dry your trousers really fast.

Aqua drying The fabric has a special membrane thing that repels water, but it won't put Moses out of a job the next time your path takes you across the Red Sea.

Equilibrium coating You'll be just as wet on the outside as you will be on the inside.

InsuDown Contains enough feathers to stuff a super king-size 38-tog duvet. When wearing InsuDown products, hikers tend to waddle, which isn't a good look.

Silver-threaded Supposedly fights bacteria to prevent unpleasant body odour. The current high price of precious metals means a stranded hiker can also melt it down in an emergency to raise urgent cash, or alternatively, make some nice earrings.

Bug bouncing Armour-plated defence against dive-bombing beasties in the Highlands.

Anything ending in 'tex' At least four times the price you think it should be. If there isn't already a brand called 'Dear-tex', there should be.

If you're trying to bamboozle enthusiasts or assistants, it's always a good idea to drop some sort of fabric into the conversation. They usually begin with 'poly' and end in 'lene', which just leaves you to think up something to go in the middle. Experience suggests that using existing fabric names to fill this gap usually works. You are unlikely to be quizzed in detail about your revolutionary new material because advances in technology mean that new fabrics are launched everyday.

'Hi, I'm looking for an outer-layer coat made from the new poly-cotton-denim-lene. Do you have any in stock?'

Such a query should cause the shop assistant's eyes to glaze over briefly as he realises that he should have been paying attention during the staff meeting earlier. Don't get too cocky, though. The shop assistant will quickly recover from this by eagerly suggesting a different material – which is probably fictitious too. But treasure that brief moment when you had the upper hand.

Footwear

There was a time when hikers could only buy one type of hiking boot: a huge clodhopper of a thing that weighed more than twice their own body weight, took six years to 'break in' and mould to their feet, and only caused blisters when there was a vowel in the month.

Things have changed. Not only do today's boots feel like slippers as soon as you slip them on, but they can be three-season or four-season, lightweight, fabric, breathable, and come with anti-clogging soles or traction control.

This makes life difficult.

Walk into an outdoor gear shop and ask for a pair of 'ordinary walking boots' and the red flashing lights with foghorn sirens will erupt telling everyone within a 50-mile radius that you are a complete greenhorn. A few minutes getting up to speed on the technicalities should save you from discomfort of both kinds.

Crampons Not excruciating calf pains that cause you to leap out of bed screaming in agony, but an additional contraption for extreme winter hiking. These vicious-looking metal spikes strap on to your boots, enabling you to trek across snow and ice – the hiking equivalent of snow chains for car tyres. If you're going hiking in such conditions, you will need a sturdier and more solidly constructed boot made from thicker leather, often referred to as a four-season boot. Start talking crampons and the outdoor gear shop assistants will respect you. Only nutters like them go out hiking on snow.

Three-season boots Self-explanatory. If you have the good sense to stay in the pub in winter, you'll need only three-season boots. The idea is that they keep your feet dry and secure for at least nine months of the year.

Fabric Lightweight boots for lightweight hikers.

Walking shoes An ordinary shoe with a beefed-up rubber sole. More for show than getting dirty and negotiating harsh terrain. The hiking equivalent of a Chelsea tractor.

Walking sandals Useful for hiking along beaches, they tend to be worn as a fashion statement – unless of course, walking socks are worn at the same time, in which case you may as well put the anorak on, too.

Nubuck leather Rawhide leather that has been brushed to give it a velvet-effect look. The velvety appearance is unlikely to survive a peat bog.

Like outdoor clothing, walking boots now come with technological buzzwords for the bluffer to be aware of, should they not want the ground from under their feet to be swept away by a particularly knowledgeable outdoor gear shop assistant.

Memory foam insoles Insoles that mould to your feet, making your boots uncomfortable for other people to wear.

Air cushioning Feels like you're walking on air, which could happen if you're traversing Striding Edge and you take a step too far. Note that this particular knife-edge ridge on Helvellyn is a useful 'favourite hike' for bluffers to drop into conversation.

Anti-clogging soles Prevent you from carrying most of the farmer's field you've just crossed on the rest of your walk. This also prevents ankle injuries caused by wheel spin when clogged soles come into contact with wet grass.

EVA (ethylene vinyl acetate) Provides cushioning comfort in the soles. Also offers rebounding benefits, literally pushing your foot back into the air, ready for the next step. Too much EVA can feel like walking on two pogo sticks.

Hiking boots are one of the most important purchases a hiker can make. Following these simple steps when making a purchase will convince any outdoor gear shop assistant that you know exactly what you're doing. And this, of course, is every bluffer's aim.

1. Buy boots in the morning. Feet swell during the day, so the earlier in the day you buy boots, the better they will fit.
2. Wear the socks you would normally wear when going hiking. Not only does this help you find boots that fit, it means you don't have to wear those spare socks that hiking shops have for the amateurs who forget such important points. Wearing other people's hiking socks is like wearing other people's underwear: not recommended.
3. Search for a hiking shop with a decent incline board – these are designed to help you test how the boots

feel when walking up- and downhill. Angled at about 45°, many are no more than 46cm (18 inches) long, leaving you with no option but to stand on them and try not to fall off. By the way, never grab the shoulder of an assistant or hiking companion. All hikers, accustomed as they are to crossing sharp, rocky ledges, are supposed to have a natural sense of balance.

ß

A hiker always has four-season walking boots, crampons, a survival bag and a two-week supply of dried food – and that's just when going to collect the morning newspaper.

VITAL EQUIPMENT

Telling the difference between each grade of walker is relatively easy. The more dedicated a walker is, the more technical the equipment. An ambler, for example, wears slippers and smokes a pipe, whereas a hiker always has four-season walking boots, crampons, a survival bag and a two-week supply of dried food – and that's just when going to collect the morning newspaper.

A bluffer should always aim to look like a hiker, even if he or she is really an ambler at heart.

Novices tend to think that all you need in order to hike is a good pair of feet and some legs that work. They certainly help, but dedicated hikers also need the right stuff in order to navigate their way back home. Getting lost (or being temporarily misplaced) is so much more dignified if you can blame it on a poorly designed piece of equipment.

GPS SATELLITE NAVIGATION

With all those satellites floating above the earth, it is possible to use a GPS device to help you navigate. These work by searching for the nearest satellites and then measuring the time taken for a signal to travel between the two. From that, they can calculate your position.

The system was developed by the US military to improve the accuracy of long-range missiles and other artillery. Initially, the accuracy of the system for hikers and other civilians was to within 10m (33ft), but this is improving all the time, which is of particular benefit to hikers following cliff paths when a sea mist has rolled in.

The US system of satellites is called Navstar, the Russians have Glonass, and not to be outdone, the European Union version is called Galileo.

In the early days of GPS, many sceptical hikers often teased those who used the devices – mainly because if a hiker walked through a dense canopy of trees, the device was no longer capable of finding the satellites it needed to calculate a location. Today, such receivers are far more sophisticated, and many smartphones now have built-in GPS receivers.

Bluffers using their smartphone GPS unit should always get out a paper map when encountering other hikers in order to show off their traditional map-reading skills. Remember to turn down the volume on your smartphone or the next instruction to 'Turn right at the spitting llama' will expose you.

Of course, all parties agree that a GPS device is only useful if the batteries aren't flat.

RUCKSACKS

Rucksacks now come in two varieties: daysacks and backpacks. Women can get away with wearing a daysack: small, delicate affairs with room inside to carry the merest of basic equipment for a short hike around the local common (mobile phone, replacement make-up, emergency chocolate bar, emergency nail file, emergency tweezers – in fact, anything they like as long as they qualify the item with the word 'emergency'). Many female hikers feel they are going back to basics with a daysack, and might feel a little vulnerable without a handbag the size of a buffalo.

Hikers whose rucksacks pull them over backwards don't get very far, rather like tortoises.

Backpacks can be equally huge. Confusingly, to the uninitiated, their capacity is measured in litres. Between 30 and 50 litres is large enough for most day hikes; anything over 50 litres and you can take your entire wardrobe with you. Hikers in the know go for good, supportive hip straps, as they carry most of the weight around their waist rather than hanging it from their shoulders. However, hip straps are notoriously difficult to control when the rucksack is standing on the floor. They are excellent at tripping people up in the pub or at coach stations. Of course, you could use this to your advantage if you want to snare someone you fancy. …

Sadly, rucksacks are not always waterproof. They should be lined with thick plastic survival bags if you want to stop your loo roll from disintegrating. They also have a tendency to pull the wearer over backwards. Hikers whose rucksacks pull them over backwards don't get very far, rather like tortoises.

Serious hikers (and well-prepared bluffers) often purchase a wire net with a padlock to chain their rucksack to a drainpipe or other immovable object when they need to leave it unattended. This is particularly useful at the start of a hike when the contents have not yet acquired the strong, sweaty odour that normally automatically repels opportunistic thieves.

WALKING POLES

Finding a fallen tree branch to use as a walking stick might seem romantic, but nature rarely drops branches that are straight, of an optimum height, or in the right place. Walking poles avoid this by being dead straight and height-adjustable, and the wise hiker will opt to use one.

Each pole reduces the strain and stress on the knees and legs by 25%, so hikers using two poles benefit from a 50% strain reduction, which means that longer distances can be covered. Sadly, using four poles does not reduce strain by 100%. Hard-core hikers do it with poles.

SUNGLASSES

Many hikers wouldn't be seen dead without their sunglasses on. The fact that the lenses are sometimes so dark that they can't see the cliff edge means that they may die happy.

WATER BOTTLE/SYSTEM

Water bottles now come in a variety of manly shapes. Alternatively, you may raise your status by using an inbuilt hydration system. It consists of a bladder bag that slips neatly into a rucksack, and all that can be seen is a long plastic tube stretching over your shoulder to your mouth. It maintains a consistent weight, because what you suck from one bladder merely trickles into your other bladder.

Hydration systems are perfect for hikers without friends. Sociable hikers simply ask their companions to get their water bottle out of their rucksacks for them, so they don't have to take them off their backs. Even in company, a hydration system ensures a water supply to yourself; hikers may share hip flasks, but they *never* suck on each other's tubes.

WATER FILTERS

Never fill your water bottle from the fast-flowing, cool waters of that crystal-clear mountain stream. It may look idyllic as it drops over the rocks in a pure and refreshing way, but the dead sheep rotting half a mile upstream will ensure that you remember your hike for many days to come. Water filters enable you to work up your own sweat as you pump the stream water ferociously through the microscopic filters, producing less pure water than you've just lost.

TORCHES

These help you study the map when your afternoon hike takes a little bit longer than expected.

PENKNIFE

Penknives come with nail files, corkscrews, bottle openers and a long, thin, pointy thing for getting stones out of horses' hooves. They'd be more useful if they had a built-in mobile-phone charger or a quick-brew tea-making facility.

FIRST-AID KITS

Life on the hills can be dangerous, which means that a basic first-aid kit with bandages, antiseptic wipes, suture and needle kits, painkillers, plasters, latex gloves and insect repellent should be carried at all times. Defibrillators may be taking things too far. Always keep a spare £20 note in your first-aid kit. It is useful in an emergency situation when you discover that your walking companions have all accidentally left their wallets behind, and it's your turn to buy the next round of drinks.

PEDOMETERS/FITNESS TRACKERS

Never wear a pedometer or a fitness tracker. Seasoned hikers know how far they've walked just by smelling the air. (The further the walk, the more pungent the body odour.) Pedometers work by measuring movement and are usually worn on a belt around the hips to record the 'shock' vibrations in the hip when the foot hits the ground. They are notoriously inaccurate because they are reliant on hikers entering their average stride length.

Fitness trackers worn on the wrist use three-axis accelerometers (a good bluffer's term, so commit it to memory) to track movement in any direction. This data is processed and used to calculate the number of steps taken, and how many calories you've burned. Some use light technology to measure your pulse, although the results aren't always as precise as one might like. Indeed, seeing your heartrate flatlining is enough to give many hikers a heart attack in itself.

Not only do inexperienced walkers with pedometers spend all their time looking at their devices and not where they're going, but they soon realise that a pedometer's recording ability improves with violent hip-swinging action. Pedometer-wearing novices wiggle their hips aggressively.

Hikers with fitness trackers spend a similar amount of time looking at their wrist display, chuffed at the 50 calories they've burned over the last eight miles, completely disregarding the 2,900 calories they've just consumed in the pub. Dishonest hikers up their step-rate simply by sitting down and waving their arm in the air.

FOOD

Successful hiking is all about successful food management. Think of your body as a steam engine and the food as the coal your body burns to produce fuel. There is an axiom that recommends that people should breakfast like a king, lunch like a lord and dine like a pauper. You are encouraged to throw this out, along with one-inch to one-mile maps. You should aim to breakfast like a hiker, lunch like a hiker, and snack like a hiker, all before dining like a hiker when your walk is done.

Breakfast This should consist of the biggest, fattiest fry-up you can muster. There will be plenty of time to worry about your cholesterol when you get back to work.

Elevenses To be taken any time after breakfast. If eaten immediately after breakfast there is less weight to carry in your rucksack.

Lunch All hikers eat at country pubs. It's the reason for going on a hike in the first place.

Afternoon snack A pick-me-up during the afternoon is a hiking necessity.

Dinner After hiking a long distance, you deserve a hearty meal, but the volume of food you want to consume may alarm non-hikers. The best course of action is to book an early table at 7pm in one restaurant, and a 9pm table at a different one. You will also benefit from a wider choice of menu and dining companions.

YOU'LL NEVER WALK ALONE

GROUP THERAPY OR ROAM ALONE?

If you wish to experience the great outdoors without having to worry about little details like navigation, you are advised to seek out other walkers. The benefits include:

* someone else to do the map reading so you can admire the view without having to stop and check where you're going
* other people to chat to
* plenty of people to carry you if you trip and break a leg
* a comfy coach to pick you up at the other end.

There are a few negative points that should be considered, which may encourage you to roam alone instead.

* You have to stick with the group and can't go explore another, more inviting-looking path.
* Crossing stiles can take time, especially if the group is a large one. Hours can be wasted if you meet a similar group coming in the other direction.
* Hiking leaders always underestimate a route's length. 'It's only 8km (five miles); my 89-year-old great-aunt could do it', may be a slight deviation from the truth.
* You're guaranteed to be the one who gets stuck with the group bore (who's still recovering from a nasty graze on his big toe and really wants to share the details with you).

GUIDEBOOKS

Guidebooks are for timid hikers: those who like to have their hands held as they walk. Phrases like 'Turn left at the third daffodil' or 'Cross the field towards the lone tree in the middle before bearing right to the stile opposite' lull the reader into a false sense of security. That's not exploring the great open countryside; that's being chauffeur-driven. In any case, Sod's Law says that the day the book is published is the day that lone tree is struck by lightning and turned to cinders.

Rumour has it that farmers buy a lot of hiking guidebooks and then go out and swap all the wooden gates on their land for metal ones, just to confuse the reader. Either that, or they sell the field to a property developer who then builds a housing estate on it. Whatever the case, to be effective, it's imperative that the bluffer uses only the guidebooks dedicated hikers keep in their rucksacks. These are the *Wainwright Pictorial Guides*.

Alfred Wainwright is revered as the patron saint of hikers. His hand-drawn guides were produced in the 1950s and 1960s and subsequently updated (even they have not escaped the march of time and the subsequent erosion of sheep pens and stone walls).

What establishes Wainwright above every other guidebook writer is that he doesn't tell you by which route to climb a hill; he tells you of several, then lets you decide which one to take. When you've made that decision, he takes the opportunity to describe what the experience is like, to marvel at the views, to wonder at the cragginess of the rocks and the sounds of the water gurgling between the rocks. These are the comments of a true hiker.

Bluffers cannot go wrong if overheard uttering a few choice Wainwright phrases. His most famous quote relates to Innominate Tarn on his favourite Lakeland ascent, Haystacks. It was there that he wanted his ashes to be scattered:

'And if you, dear reader, should get a bit of grit in your boot as you are crossing Haystacks in the years to come, please treat it with respect. It might be me.'

GEOCACHING

The intelligent bluffer will have realised the true potential that GPS offers hikers. Not only does it give them another excuse for becoming temporarily misplaced when their batteries go flat, or when a satellite that's tracking them gets taken out by a rogue comet, it also offers them an opportunity to have some fun. And if you're going to be temporarily misplaced, you might as well have fun doing it.

Geocaching is treasure hunting for hikers, with an element of social inclusion thrown in. Instead of wandering aimlessly with a metal detector, listening for the ever-increasing frequency of beeps that denote the discovery of yet another lost Saxon hoard, hikers programme the coordinates of the treasure, obtained from one of the many geocaching websites, into their GPS system and then follow its directions to locate the treasure, or 'cache' as you should refer to it. If only Saxon hoarders had logged the global positioning coordinates of their hoards on the relevant website, treasure hunters could have saved themselves many a wet Wednesday afternoon standing in a farmer's field, hoping the beeping noise emanating from the cowpat beneath them was buried treasure and not a zip fastener dropped by a passing hiker.

For geocaching to work properly, someone needs to hide a cache somewhere discreet, and note its coordinates on their GPS device. These coordinates are then added to a geocaching website, where other geocachers can download them to their GPS devices and go out in search of the treasure.

While these coordinates help a geocacher find the right location (which could be anywhere on the planet, hence the 'geo' element of the word 'geocache'), it does not explain where the cache is hidden. And these caches can be cleverly disguised. The next time you see a hiker halfway up a tree, he might not be trying to gain altitude in an attempt to find his bearings; he could simply be looking for treasure.

Caches may be hidden in the crook of a tree, in a false stone on a pebbly beach, or even in a plastic bird set into a riverbank. They come in a variety of sizes (caches, not just plastic birds by riverbanks), and understanding the correct terminology will assist a bluffer when looking for their cache.

Micro Less than 100ml in volume. Usually an old 35mm film canister. Somebody had to find a use for those plastic tubes once we ditched celluloid and went digital with our photos.

Small More than 100ml, but less than one litre. A small plastic sandwich box. If the cache inside turns out to be a fresh salmon with caviar on a bed of micro-lettuce sandwich, then you really have found treasure. If it's before its sell-by date, even better.

Regular More than one litre, but less than 20 litres. Typically shoebox-size. Hikers get excited when the contents are a pair of boots, their size, and newer than the pair they're wearing.

Large More than 20 litres. Typically a bucket. Usually with an animal eating the cache out of it.

To sound authoritative, bluffers should remind their audience that geocaching is not about 'finders keepers'. Some caches, especially the micro-caches, are merely log sheets where geocachers record their name and the date they found the non-existent treasure. (Yes, even if there isn't any, it's still called 'treasure'.) The log sheet is more environmentally friendly than scratching 'I woz 'ere' in the bark of a tree, or gouging it into a nearby boulder. The larger caches may have items contained within them, as well as a log sheet, or logbook.

Unlike real treasure, the rule of geocaching insists that if you take something from the cache, then you must replace it with something else of equal or higher value. Over a period of many years, it presumably follows that the geocacher who originally hid the treasure could find that his or her initial treasure of a paper clip has turned into the deeds for a six-bedroom apartment, with pool, in Miami.

The advent of geocaching means that hikers have had to learn new terminology, therefore a bluffer would do well to drop some of the following terms into a conversation with a passing hiker to determine whether they are a geocaching hiker or a geo-muggle (a non-geocaching hiker):

Ground Zero This is where your GPS unit confirms you have arrived at the cache location. Your treasure is around here somewhere – assuming you haven't already trodden on it.

Hitch-hiker This refers to an item of treasure in the cache which has instructions for you to take it on to a new location. This ensures that the treasure sees more of the world than you do.

TNLN Code for 'Took Nothing, Left Nothing'. Despite treasure being available, the last geocacher recorded the successful finding of the cache, but couldn't be arsed to do anything with it. These are generally hikers who have yet to experience the real joy of geocaching.

Webcam cache At webcam caches there are no log sheets or books. When a geocacher finds a webcam cache they phone a friend to log on to the relevant webcam website and get them to take a picture of them standing in front of the camera, proving they found the cache. In London, the Metropolitan Police know webcam caches as CCTV.

Hikers who spot a furtive geocacher surreptitiously hiding a cache should smile and shout: 'Don't worry: I won't claim FTF status!' Using this term (First to Find) demonstrates you're in the know about geocaching and will not call the bomb squad as one ignorant, geo-muggle did in Wetherby, West Yorkshire.

Unfortunately for that geocacher, after the police sealed off the street, a unit of the Royal Logistic Corps from Catterick Garrison wheeled out its robot to initiate a controlled explosion. Instead of being in one location, the geocache was now in hundreds of tiny pieces, scattered across the entire street. Had each piece been left where it was, its coordinates could have been taken to create what's known as a multi-cache geocache. This enables geocachers to follow a trail of coordinates, each offering a clue to the next location, eventually revealing a grand cache.

Some may be forgiven for thinking that all of hiking's effects on health are beneficial. While the overall effect is good, the maxim 'no pain – no gain' will come to mind. So prepare yourself for the pain.

HEALTH AND SAFETY

A Japanese theory states that if you walk 10,000 steps a day you will maintain your current weight, and if you do more than 10,000 steps a day, you will lose weight. The lesson here is not to take too many steps in one day; otherwise you may lose so much weight that you disappear completely.

Hiking is supposed to be healthy. Not only is it one of the best all-round workouts you can give your body, it can also improve your mental state. More and more GPs advise taking a daily 30-minute walk for those who are down in the dumps. Of course, it could be based on a misunderstanding. When the 48th patient of the day walks into the surgery and says 'I'm depressed'. he may well be told to take a hike.

However, you will recall that walking stimulates the human brain to secrete endorphins, a natural form of painkiller that resembles opium-derived drugs such as morphine and heroin. This is why hikers enjoy hiking so much. It's all about being spaced out. When hikers talk about the high they get at the top of a mountain, it has nothing to do with altitude.

Some may be forgiven for thinking that all the effects on health are beneficial. You will know better. While the overall effect is good, the maxim 'no pain – no gain' will come to mind.

So prepare yourself for the pain.

BLISTERS

This is what happens when something rubs you up the wrong way (except close relatives, of course). Blisters are the bane of many a hiker's life because they can be immensely painful and ruin a good day out. The only way to recover is to rest, which is no use whatsoever if you still have 15 miles to go to get back to the car.

If walking boots are the wrong size, or too loosely laced, they'll rub against the socks and skin. As soon as you feel a blister developing, stop walking and take your boots and socks off. Scrutinise your feet, looking for the offending, fluid-filled growth, and then ask yourself the all-important question: to burst or not to burst?

If out with other hikers, ask their opinion, then go with the minority decision stating, 'It's surprising there doesn't seem to be any right treatment for this common ailment.' Hardened hikers are divided into 'bursters' or 'patchers'.

A burster will free the gunge building up inside. Should you be lucky enough to have a long, pointy thing for getting stones out of horses' hooves on your penknife, this is ideal. Bursting can reduce the pain and allow your foot to recover more quickly. However, as patchers often point out, you run an increased risk of infection. To avoid this, apply a sterile membrane (which you will always carry in your backpack). Hiking becomes more difficult if you lose a foot due to gangrene.

Patchers take a more softly, softly approach. They apply a piece of cushioning material over the distressed area to act as a barrier and prevent any further friction. This can be anything from the first-aid kit – a plaster, a piece of gauze and some tape, or a bit of bandage.

Hiking becomes more difficult if you lose a foot due to gangrene.

A patcher will ask, 'What's the point of bursting the blister if you end up doing what patchers prefer doing, and covering the painful area with a protective membrane?'

There are several products on the market that provide a high-tech solution to the problem. Real hikers never use them, so the bluffer should do so discreetly, if at all.

The sensible way to treat blisters is to avoid them in the first place. Always:

*   Wear good hiking socks. Seamless are best because there are no seams to rub against your feet. Darning just isn't an option. Rumours that hikers should change their socks on a daily basis are false. Any hiker knows that it takes four days for a sock to

mould itself to the foot, thereby creating the perfect fit. So always make sure that you have the right sock on the right foot.

* Tie laces tightly enough to prevent your boots from rubbing. If that means a double knot under your chin, then so be it.

* As hard skin prevents blisters, walk about barefoot before going for a hike.

* Remove any foreign bodies you find in your socks. Tell them to buy their own.

SPRAINS

Spraining your ankle is painful. After the pain of tearing ligaments comes the swelling. Don't expect instant recovery – it can take up to six weeks – and serious sprains may require surgery. Reduce the swelling with ice which, naturally, you have brought with you in a thermos or chilly container for just such a contingency. You can't rely on there being a cold mountain stream nearby when you crick an ankle.

SUNBURN

Not only does the physical activity of hiking release endorphins in your brain, hiking in sunshine can increase their number. The risk of sunburn is that much greater, particularly if you're 914m (3,000ft) up a mountain. It stands to reason: you're closer to the sun.

Always wear a high-factor suncream and apply it

often. This is useful for bluffers just beginning their hiking experiences, because it gives them an additional excuse to stop for a rest. And don't forget that hat: the wider the brim the better. But draw the line at sombreros.

CHAFING

Chafing is like blisters. The cause is the same – friction generated by something rubbing against the body – only in more embarrassing places. Armpits, shoulders, legs and the groin areas are most common. For many hikers, lubrication is the best solution, with petroleum jelly being the favoured choice. Always apply your own, never anyone else's. Reaching the bottom of your left shoulder blade may not be easy, and the temptation to ask for help is great, but be aware that you might be asked to reciprocate. And you can never tell where their affected area might be.

BITERS

The great outdoors is a dangerous place, and the bluffer should be aware of this. Sometimes the countryside doesn't like you traipsing all over it, and it bites back. Your attackers include the following:

Horseflies
Unlike other bloodsuckers, which stick thin needles in you and suck out your life-source, horseflies rip your flesh apart and then have a feast. This is why horsefly

'bites' are more painful than others. The females are the ones you have to watch out for because they do the feasting. However, it is a rare bluffer who can identify the gender of a horsefly.

Midges

The Scottish Highland midge is one of the fiercest of the 40 or so species of biting midge. They are attracted by the carbon dioxide that humans breathe out. With a wingspan of less than 2mm they don't take huge chunks out of hikers' arms, but the bite is enough to cause itching and swelling for several days.

Midges prefer gang warfare. You will rarely be bitten only once and are more likely to be attacked by an entire squadron. Global warming is encouraging these annoying biters to invade other areas of the UK, including the Lake District and North Wales. There are four steps to avoiding midges:

1. Learn to love the DEET invisible cloak. Most midge repellents use this chemical because it blocks the insect's ability to detect you. It's like wearing the Harry Potter invisible cloak, without being invisible.
2. Buy a midge hat with netting that covers your face – ideal for hikers who like the funereal look. Ensure that you don't trap a midge in there with you, though.
3. Seek out the Midge Forecast, often published in Scottish newspapers, or download the Midge Forecast app for your smartphone.
4. Stop breathing out.

Ticks

Related to scorpions and spiders, ticks live in damp, vegetative conditions (woodlands, bracken and long grass) particularly where sheep and deer are found. Latching on to passing flesh, ticks often start off the size of a pinhead but as their blood sac fills, they swell to the size of a pea – yet you are usually completely unaware that you've been bitten.

Ticks are tenacious. Getting rid of one is as difficult as escaping the clutches of an outdoor gear shop assistant keen to make a sale. Never hold it by its blood sac (the tick, not the shop assistant) and pull. This could simply force the tick to regurgitate your blood, and any disease it is currently harbouring, back into your own blood supply. The worst gift it can give you is Lyme disease. Remove by grasping close to its embedded mouth parts and pulling out straight. If you find a bit still left, pull it out, too. Better still, avoid ticks by employing these techniques:

1. Tuck your trousers into your socks – not a great fashion statement, but evidence that you are tick-aware.
2. Splash some DEET on exposed surfaces – it covers up that carbon dioxide smell.
3. Reapply DEET regularly.

Adders

Britain's only poisonous snakes will, on average, bite 100 people every year, although in the UK there have only been 14 deaths caused by adder bites since 1876, the last in 1975. The biggest risk is from anaphylactic shock. The next is being allergic to the antivenom. You can easily identify an adder by the black zigzag markings on its skin, and should walk away carefully if you spot one. Most snakebites result from disturbing or picking up an adder – although why anyone would wish to pick up a poisonous snake is something of a mystery.

If you are in the company of someone who gets bitten, try to raise the bitten part of the body high in the air. Do not be tempted to suck out the venom, Indiana Jones-style, because it could be accidentally swallowed. In any case, there are parts of a fellow hiker's body at which even the most compassionate bluffer might draw a line.

Seek medical attention immediately and start praying, even if you're not religious.

MOUNTAIN RESCUE

While you might hold the understandable view that hikers who go out in all weathers are a bit unhinged, you will appreciate that there is one exception: members of the intrepid Mountain Rescue services. These include the RAF which will airlift you off a mountain should you break a leg, twist an ankle, or become trapped by bad weather; plus the brave, unpaid volunteers of the Mountain Rescue teams on the ground. Both are on call 24 hours a day, 7 days a week, every day of the year – for emergencies.

An emergency is something that is life-threatening. Unfortunately, needing help to get back to level ground in time to catch your train doesn't qualify. Hinting that you might once have been a member of the Mountain Rescue services is a good bluff, but never overplay it. In fact resolutely refuse to discuss it further, saying something like: 'If you've seen *Touching the Void,* you'll understand why I don't want to talk about it.' Striking a noble pose, firm-jawed, with a faraway look in the eye is recommended in these circumstances.

FELL TOP ASSESSORS

You are strongly advised to grasp the hand of a fell top assessor warmly should you come face to face with one while hiking in the Lake District. A fell top assessor is not someone who scores every mountain summit out of ten for the scenic quality of its views, as some might think, although should you stop to chat to one, he or she will no doubt share with you a most memorable vista. Assessors actually perform a vital role in ensuring a safe hiking environment. Every time you ring the Lake District's Weatherline (0844 846 2444), not only will you receive Met Office weather forecasting for climbing Lakeland's mountains, but the information will also be augmented by the findings of a fell top assessor.

These are some of the most dedicated hikers in the country (although most less dedicated hikers might think they need sectioning). Between December and March, a fell top assessor climbs to the summit of Helvellyn, England's third-highest mountain (950m or 3,117ft), every day.

Correct: *they climb to the summit of the same mountain every day for four months.*

Once up there, they take a few photos, lick their finger and stick it in the air to assess wind direction, record what the weather conditions are like, and then make their way back down again.

You'll need to know why they are climbing only the third-highest mountain in England, and not the highest, Scafell Pike (978m or 3,209ft). The reason is that Helvellyn's large, wall-like east face means that it maintains snow on its summit for longer than its taller Lakeland sister, making it the more dangerous summit for wintry weather conditions.

And hikers always need to know the degree of risk before they set out (if they've got any sense).

CLOSE ENCOUNTERS (OF THE HERD KIND)

Properly equipped, you should by now be capable of tackling the freedom of the open footpath. However, the problem with the right to roam and the desire to tramp the hills without hindrance is that, once you remove the restrictions, it is not only hikers who can roam. Sheep can do it, too. To stop them straying too far, farmers build fences and walls and dig deep ditches. A hike thus becomes a full-blown obstacle course.

STILES

Very few hikers can negotiate a stile gracefully, so don't even bother trying.

Traditional stiles are constructed from wood in a fence shape, with a plank supported on both sides to be used as a step. Sometimes tall stiles have two planks, offering two steps on either side. Never let the sight of more than one step lull you into a false sense of security, particularly if you're male. The genital-preserving technique that all hardened hikers use is to ensure that the distance between the top of the highest step and the top of the stile is less than their inside leg measurement. Failure to do so could result in one singing 'The Happy Wanderer' several octaves higher at the end of the walk than at the beginning.

Ladder stiles are used to negotiate taller boundaries, such as deer fencing or tall stone walls, and require the hiker to climb up to 3m (10ft) off the ground. This frequently sends hikers into a fearful tizzy because:

* Despite the fact that they enjoy climbing mountains of over 914m (3,000ft), climbing above the third rung of a ladder can still set off a chronic bout of vertigo.
* The top of a ladder stile is often exposed, meaning hikers with large rucksacks are prone to being blown to the other side of the valley by a rogue gust of wind.
* They often lead to arguments about how to descend the other side: by turning around and facing the ladder, or walking down the rungs as if they were a set of stairs. Experienced hikers always turn around and face the ladder for a secure descent. Those who treat them like stairs frequently slip, falling face-first into the inevitably waiting cowpat. Admittedly, this can be hugely entertaining.

Those of you with a technical bent will remember to add an extra allowance when calculating the total ascent and descent of a walk to take into account the number of ladder stiles encountered en route.

KISSING GATES

Like hikers, these come in all shapes and sizes – with one exception. They do *not* cater for the obese (they're never big enough). A hinged gate swings between two enclosed points – hence the 'kiss' as it makes contact with each end of the enclosure. Those who come across such contraptions for the first time should watch a more experienced hiker tackle this mechanism first to learn how not to use it.

Always observe from a distance.

Note how the hiker approaches the gate and pushes it away, revealing a small enclosure to one side, into which he or she steps, backing into it as far as possible. In theory, the hiker should now be able to pull the gate right back, to 'kiss' the other point, creating a gap large enough to allow passage into the next field. This theory is based upon three points:

1. The gate hinges allow full and free movement, permitting the gate to swing to its full arc.
2. The hiker is a size zero (or even thinner than that if wearing a large rucksack).
3. The hiker coming in the opposite direction isn't blocking the exit.

Landowners who want to inflict pain upon anyone passing through the kissing gates can enhance them with 'add-ons'. Attaching coiled springs to the hinges allows them to swing back with enough force to crush the knuckles of any following hiker whose hand is resting on the gated area. In bleak areas, instead of springs, landowners sometimes use a large boulder or cement block, wrap a chain around it, and tie one end to the gate, the other to the fence. It's the weight of the boulder that keeps the gate closed. For the hiker, extra force is required to open the gate in the first place. As soon as the grip on the gate is released, gravity takes over. The gate slams shut against the knuckles of the hiker behind, while at the same time the boulder plummets to the ground, crushing his or her foot.

It can be tough out there in the great outdoors.

BLOCKAGES

Amateurs tend to think that hikers spend all day wandering freely among the hills. In fact, while wandering free of charge is possible (apart from exorbitant parking charges), wandering unhindered isn't as easy as some might think. Blockages can occur almost anywhere, and encountering a hiker with a pained expression will usually mean that the root of the problem lies with a blockage. (Anyone encountering a hiker with a pained expression and partially obscured behind a tree should make themselves scarce. There are some types of blockage that other hikers just do not wish to know about.)

The joy and the frustration of hiking is that the surroundings may change on a daily basis. What was a clear path yesterday may today be completely blocked by a tangle of intertwined vegetation fed by seven hours of continuous rain overnight. As your equipment usually doesn't include several pounds' worth of explosives or a flamethrower, you may have to fall back on an appropriate tool in your Swiss Army knife (the falling back should be figurative, not literal). The alternative to clearing a blockage is simply to walk around the offending item, but this can take time. The worst blockages are the size of entire cities.

Landowners who do not appreciate hikers crossing their land may decide to install their own blockages. This is illegal, and hikers can take action to clear the offending material – although moving several large canisters of highly toxic substances is best left to the experts.

A survey has revealed that hikers find their right of way blocked on a third of all the walks they undertake. You are therefore recommended to use the other two-thirds of rights of way, which are clear and problem-free. If you don't complete a hike and want to save face, invent a suitable blockage.

ELECTRIC FENCES

Electric fences add a certain frisson of excitement to a walk. Landowners are entitled to use electric fencing near, alongside and across rights of way on a temporary basis, especially if it helps them to keep their livestock in check. Some landowners have realised that electric fencing also keeps hikers in check.

If an electric fence crosses a right of way, a safe means of crossing the fence should be made available. This usually involves covering the electrified wire with some insulating material, which is generally no more than a bit of old rag or a dead mole. It tends to be hikers with short inside-leg measurements who most fear crossing electric fences, although there is a masochistic band of walkers who take pleasure in crossing such power-charged boundaries. It is impossible to explain why.

The responsible farmer or landowner will identify an electric fence by displaying suitable warning signs at every 25m (82ft) interval. These may depict the outline of a person being struck by lightning, which is a nice touch.

Alternatively, the bottom of the fence line might be littered with the charred carcasses of small dead animals, some of which can serve as additional insulation (*see* above).

WAYMARKS

Waymarks are for wimps, and signposts are for softies. Expert hikers always know which way to go, and usually it's any way they like.

A waymark is traditionally a small plastic disc with a coloured arrow on it, reputedly pointing in the rough direction of the right of way. Novice hikers can be easily identified because they are often seen consulting their maps and looking up at the sky. They are not fazed by left- or right-pointing waymarks, but a waymark indicating 'straight on' usually points 'straight up'. Put them out of their misery by telling them that the path upwards is blocked by a particularly nasty cumulonimbus cloud and should be avoided at all costs.

Traditionally, waymarks are nailed to solid objects that will not move for a while, including:

* stiles
* gateposts
* tree trunks
* boulders or stones
* dead sheep

Local authorities and landowners enjoy playing games with hikers, the most popular of which is called 'hunt the waymark'. They have perfected the skill of hiding such directional aids in the depths of flesh-tearing hedges, which prevent well-clad hikers from investigating further for fear of ripping their expensive outdoor clothing. There is little point in buying something with space-age technology if a simple thorn can render the garment completely useless.

By law, all rights of way should be signposted where they meet a road or public highway. Camouflaging them enables the landowner and local authority to comply with the letter of the law, while making it difficult for ramblers to exercise their right to roam.

Some kindly authorities cater for the new hiker just starting out on the long journey of discovery by spelling out the type of right of way they are on. Bluffers may come across helpful signs declaring 'Public Footpath' or 'Public Bridleway'. Some landowners like to show their sense of humour by installing their own signs declaring: 'I don't demand money for accessing this field, but the bull charges.' There is no law against this.

Local authorities also use a colour-coding system for the directional arrows on waymarks. For footpaths, they use yellow; blue arrows identify bridleways, which are open to cyclists and horse riders; BOATs and RUPPs (*see* pages 29–31) are marked with red arrows, possibly to signify that as motor vehicles also use these routes, hikers are taking a risk.

This system, of course, is of no use whatsoever to colour-blind hikers.

A good general rule is to beware of anything with horns.

Bluffers spotting plain white circular discs along the route should exercise extreme caution. This phenomenon occurs when the waymark is exposed to excess sunlight for prolonged periods of time (admittedly, unusual in Britain). The advice in these circumstances is to proceed quickly in order not to suffer the same consequences.

LIVESTOCK

Another joy of hiking is experiencing close encounters with the other flora and fauna with which we share this planet. Hiking provides rare opportunities to get up close and personal with creatures many other people just don't see – and to appreciate the power behind a ton of bovine muscle when it is charging at a rapidly increasing speed from a rapidly decreasing distance.

The chances of encountering livestock while out hiking are relatively high, and all bluffers should learn how to deal with each kind of animal in order to survive to tell the tale. A good general rule is to beware of anything with horns. Bulls, cows, deer, rams, or 44-ton lorries taking such animals to slaughter, should be avoided at all costs. Treat them as a blockage and look for a diversion.

Cows and bulls

Always check before you cross a field of cows to make sure that it actually is a field of cows. If the 'cow' appears to have only one udder, take the alternative footpath, even if it involves using a frayed rope to cross a bottomless ravine. It will be safer.

If these one-uddered cows are quite small, the braver hiker may risk crossing the field. These are bullocks, or young bulls. They are not real men yet; just the equivalent of teenage hoodies. They may come running towards you because they've learned about safety in numbers and know that group action frightens most humans. You should have confidence, especially if you're trying to convince your companions that you're an experienced hiker. Walking tall and proud and straight ahead will unnerve them, and eventually they'll let you through. What these hoodies fear most is an ASBO – A Supermarket Buying Order.

Of course, at this teenage stage, their parents just can't control them, and have no desire to. When the bovine offspring are much younger, a parent will always protect them. A field full of calves may look cute and picturesque, but it's the mothers you have to watch out for. They will gang up and encircle the creature they believe to be most vulnerable.

This is likely to be you.

Reach your destination by learning the language. 'Shoo!' is very rude in cattle circles, and many cows will take two steps back out of shock.

It is a myth that the colour red inflames a bull. Either that or outdoor gear manufacturers enjoy a good joke, seeing that most of their products come in shades of red. The important thing to remember is that you should always be nearer to the fence than the bull is. Should the beast decide to charge, you're more likely to reach the fence before it reaches you.

Bulls from the following breeds that are more than 10 months old are banned from fields with rights of way passing through them: Ayrshire, British Friesian, British Holstein, Dairy Shorthorn, Guernsey, Jersey and Kerry. But if a bull is charging, you will be unlikely to want to hang around to make a positive identification of the breed in question.

Sheep

There are two kinds of sheep: those that wet themselves in fear at the sight of a walker, and those that think you are a farmer and have food to offer. The first lot empty their bladders then run away. The second lot come running up and start nosing in your pockets for anything edible. Handkerchiefs, compasses, car keys and wallets are all edible to a sheep. Don't try to be funny by shouting 'Mint sauce!' It doesn't work; sheep have no sense of humour.

Horses

Horses only get aggressive when their foals are nearby. Don't even bother running in the opposite direction to jump the fence or hedge if you find yourself being chased. If you can clear the hedge, you can be sure that the horse can too.

Llamas and alpacas

These are becoming an increasingly common sight, and are often used by farmers and smallholders to protect other animals, particularly sheep and chickens. They can spit, but only if provoked, so bluffers are advised not to spit at them first.

Farm dogs

Farm gates have never seen a can of oil in their life, and do not need one. As soon as you think about sliding the latch, the noise of metal against metal is enough to alert all farm dogs within an 80km (50-mile) radius. Dogs are highly trained and know exactly which gate the hiker is using, and they will hurl themselves towards it. All 220 of them. (Farmers never have one dog. That would be a pet, and these are not pets, but working animals.)

Whether you make it to the other side of the farm depends on the age and speed of the dogs. And your own. A prudent bluffer should:

* Refrain from offering them food – your shapeless cheese and tomato sandwiches won't feed all of them and you will only encourage demands for more.
* Bark out a sergeant-style command using the word 'SIT!' and hope for the best.
* Extend a hand as a clenched fist and offer them the back of it to sniff. Once they've smelled your fear, they will do one of two things: jump up at you because you're a pushover, or run off to tell another 219 dogs to come and hassle you further.

OTHER HIKERS

From time to time, you will encounter other hikers en route. In popular areas such as the Lake District or the mountains of Snowdonia, the paths can seem as populated as a garden centre on a bank holiday Monday. There is an etiquette to acknowledging other hikers.

* Always say 'Morning!' no matter what time of day it is. This demonstrates that you are enjoying your freedom so much you are completely unaware of time passing.
* Follow on with a 'Lovely day for it, isn't it?' even though they may not be able to hear you through the hailstorm and gale-force winds. For dedicated hikers, every day is a lovely day for it, no matter what the weather.
* If you stop for a chat (and it's good to swap tales), exaggerate. If you began walking at 10 o'clock in the morning, imply that you heard the dawn chorus.

If you have only walked 3km (2 miles), suggest a somewhat higher number, and at some point casually remark that you are less than halfway round. Never allow a fellow hiker to outsmart you. If they have 12 miles still to go, you still have 15.

* Swap advice. Tell them about the particularly nasty patch of stinging nettles surrounding that third stile, and they'll warn you of the farm gate with the dodgy hinge. And the 220 dogs.

There are some hikers, though, who just want to be at one with their surroundings. Alfred Wainwright was one such. He'd catch the first bus of the day into the mountains and then hike his way over a couple of ridges to catch the last bus home. On a good day he never met a soul. Not many people used public transport then either.

These solo hikers are easily spotted. They will nod in acknowledgement as they pass by, but be long gone even before you've had a chance to open your mouth. Let them go. If they'd wanted someone to talk to them, they'd have brought a friend.

If you're eating, remember that real hikers never have starters – unless they classify the first three rounds as 'starters'.

REST AND RECOVERY

CALLS OF NATURE

Observant bluffers will have realised that hiking generates the production of a range of bodily fluids, such as perspiration, which occurs when the body generates too much heat, and it's important to replenish your fluid intake regularly to counteract this. This means water, not alcoholic beverages, which are diuretics.

However, some of what goes in must come out, and at some stage hikers must seek a suitable object to hide behind while they answer what is euphemistically termed 'a call of nature'. Such an object should be tall enough and thick enough to prevent any unnecessary exposure. It would be an act of charity to point out to companions the necessity to avoid the vicinity of an electric fence, a powerful gust of wind, or a frond of stinging nettle.

Should the call of nature involve the bowels rather than the bladder, you must be prepared. This means a plastic bag, some loo roll and a small trowel. Here are some useful tips for a successful evacuation:

* Dig a hole at least 15–20cm (6–8in) deep and at least 100m (328ft) away from any watercourse, or path.
* When you have finished, place the used loo roll in the hole and burn it – although don't do this if the surrounding material is highly combustible.
* If soil variations make it impossible to dig such a hole, remove any deposits and tissue, place them in a plastic bag, tie it securely and stash it away discreetly until you find the nearest suitable receptacle.
* Do not eat curry the night before a hike.

Seasoned hikers try to train their bodies to undertake regular bowel movements at a time that is more convenient to them – when they are at a friendly inn, and moments before someone suggests that it's their round.

PUBS

Hikers are entitled to reward themselves for their efforts. Hiking expends a lot of energy and calories, and tackling the next stage of the journey will not be possible until you've replenished what you've lost. However, you should be aware that there is still an act to keep up when replenishing yourself in an idyllic country pub. Other hikers will be watching.

* Never buy a 'half' of anything. Pints, gallons and barrels are okay. Halves are out.
* Never buy bottled beer. That's what football fans drink. Real Hikers savour Real Ale.
* Order your drink as though you're a regular: 'Hi

Frank, the usual please.' If Frank is a true barman he'll pour you a pint of his most expensive beer in the hope that it will become your 'usual'. Those sitting nearby who know that Fred is not Frank will assume that you and he go back a long way, and this is what he was called at school.

* If you're eating, remember that real hikers never have starters – unless they classify the first three rounds as 'starters'.

* Never select the scampi, far less the vegetarian options. Steak and ale pie, rib-eye steak, and toad-in-the-hole are the only choices for a true hiker. Supersize anything you can.

Never buy a 'half' of anything. Pints, gallons and barrels are okay. Halves are out.

Real log fires are a quick way to dry your boots out after hiking through several hours' worth of rain. While the heat can split the leather, hardened hikers don't mind because it gives them an excuse to buy a new pair, with even more state-of-the-art technology.

Never take your boots off and place them by the fire, though. Keep them on, so the heat from your feet will help to dry them from the inside. Also bear in mind the olfactory assault on fellow patrons should you remove them.

Avoid pubs that demand that you remove your boots before entering the lounge or bar areas (for the same reason). Or prove your love of the outdoors by insisting on eating and drinking in the beer garden so that you can admire the view. True hikers sit at a picnic table in shorts and a T-shirt supping ale as a torrential downpour descends on their already soggy chips.

FIVE OF THE BEST

The cannier bluffer will have twigged that there's a close link between hiking and pubs. Indeed, the two go hand in glove, or hand round pint, as most hikers will attest.

However, while *any* public house is clearly better than a hike that has no public house within a 50-mile radius (although most dedicated hikers would think nothing of doing the extra 50 miles to reach it), there are some public houses that attract a dedicated class of hiker, and actually become the purpose of the hike. Feel free to call them 'meccas'. Clearly, for your bluff to carry any credibility you would be wise to mention some or all of the following meccas in your next fireside chat with a fellow hiker.

Indeed, a walk linking all five is what hikers call a proper afternoon's pub crawl.

Tan Hill Inn – North Yorkshire

Any bluffer wishing to provoke unadulterated envy among their hiking companions should recall the time they were snowed in at this most famous of hikers' pubs. The Tan Hill Inn is the highest public house in Britain, dispensing alcoholic refreshments at an altitude of some 525m (1,725ft), right on the doorstep of the Pennine Way national trail.

Hikers who arrived on 31 December 2009 to celebrate the New Year found themselves still toasting 2010 some three days later, due to heavy snow. Such scenes were repeated three years later, when customers were cut off from the outside world for some five days.

Allow your listeners to believe you were caught in the great 2013 snowdrifts that inspired leading supermarket Waitrose to feature the pub in its 2017 Christmas advert. For added kudos, point them to the relevant clip on YouTube and jab the screen knowingly when an indistinguishable face peers through the heavily frosted window and say, 'That bit's based on me.'

The Old Forge, Knoydart – Scottish Highlands

It's mainland Britain's remotest pub, not that that would be a problem for the hardened hiker. With no roads in or out of the hamlet of Inverie, there are only two ways to reach it: an 18-mile trek over numerous 914m (3,000ft) high Scottish mountains, or a 7-mile sea crossing from the nearest settlement of Mallaig.

Of course, all great walks should have a pub at the end of them, so you should always explain that you did the 18-mile trek to get there, then took the less-daunting 7-mile sea crossing to get back ... but not until you'd imbibed several rounds with your fellow hikers. After all, hikers are not known for having great sea legs, so a little medicinal alcohol to numb the seasickness on the return trip is a necessity.

The Royal Oak, Cardington – Shropshire

Located in the idyllic Shropshire village of Cardington ('Salop' being a county only a true hiker can locate without the need of a map), the 15th-century Royal Oak is reputedly the oldest continuously-licensed pub in the country. And so they've had plenty of practice of serving hikers.

Your standing with fellow hikers will be immeasurably enhanced if you mention that you partook of the local delicacy, Fidget Pie, on a previous visit. Make out that during a conversation with a gnarled regular, he let slip that the secret recipe, passed down from landlord to landlord, is said to include gammon and local cider. When asked for the rest of the recipe, you will set your jaw nobly and say that you swore an oath never to reveal anything further.

The Old Dungeon Ghyll – Great Langdale, Cumbria

Historically, the Old Dungeon Ghyll Hotel was where nearly every mountain climbing club in the country went to for their annual club dinner. However, that didn't stop the hotel naming their bar the Hikers' Bar. (The nearby New Dungeon Ghyll Hotel opted to call theirs the Walkers' Bar. Should anyone establish the Even Newer Dungeon Ghyll Hotel, they'll probably name theirs the Ramblers' Bar.)

Dedicated bluffers who can identify the Old Dungeon Ghyll's location on an Ordnance Survey map in Langdale at the end of the B5343 will understand the sense in appealing to hikers. The only real passing trade at this location are walkers. Thousands of them. The idiots who continue in their cars on the single-track road with few passing places will experience the joys of several one-in-four hill climbs while coming face-to-face with a coachload of Japanese tourists travelling in the opposite direction.

That's why hikers rely on their feet. Add the fact that at the Hikers' Bar there's always a roaring log fire, a welcome no matter how muddy your boots are, and some of the best local ales in the country ... what more could a bluffer want? (Apart from an appreciative audience with whom to share their hiking knowledge.)

The Old Nag's Head, Edale – Derbyshire

This Peak District pub's claim to fame is that it's the official start of the Pennine Way national trail. Bluffers will naturally point out that walking from the pub car park into the Walkers' Bar and ordering a pre-Pennine Way pint is not actually included in the official distance of 268 miles. But who's counting? Especially when a fortifying pint is involved. Non-hikers might argue that a pint before starting the walk is a little unorthodox as part of a warm-up routine. Bluffers will reason that this first section of the Pennine Way includes the second longest ascent to be found along the trail's entire route and that, therefore, any hardened hiker will know that such inclines are more effectively scaled after a couple of swift ones before they set off. And should the hiker be just a little unsteady on their feet, as everyone knows, inclines are far easier to climb if tackled in a zigzag style or side-to-side motion (sometimes on hands and knees).

The Old Nag's Head is therefore the perfectly placed walkers' pub. Non-hikers will assume that anyone wearing clean boots at the bar has yet to start their Pennine Way journey, while those with muddy boots have tackled it in the less-traditional north to south direction and are celebrating their completion.

And that, dear Bluffer, is why a bluffing hiker never cleans their walking boots.

HANGING UP YOUR BOOTS

There comes a point in every hiker's journey when it's time to hang up your walking boots and shuffle off to the even bigger hills in the sky. This truly is an adventure because neither Ordnance Survey, Harvey, nor any other map manufacturer has maps to help hikers on this particular journey. And while your soul may be exploring the heavens, no one knows for sure whether your GPS receiver will work up there, despite the fact that you will be much closer to the satellites themselves.

Non-hikers don't understand why hikers enjoy setting off on two feet in all weathers. Occasionally, a hiker might try to explain that it's because of the fresh air, getting closer to nature, exploring the countryside or finding a good country pub. A bluffer should simply answer the question with the ancient Latin phrase *Solvitur ambulando* and adopt an expression of Zen-like contemplation.

For those who didn't learn Latin, the phrase translates as 'It is solved by walking'. Non-hikers will never know what 'it' is, but when hikers hang up their boots for the last time, they'll understand everything: including why the last mile of a walk is always four times longer than the other miles on the same route.

There's no point in pretending that you know everything about hiking – nobody does – but if you've got this far and you've absorbed at least a modicum of the information and advice contained within these pages, then you will almost certainly know more than 99% of the rest of the human race about what it involves, how it can be good for your health, why it can be bad for your feet, and how you can pretend to be more knowledgeable about it than you are.

What you now do with this information is up to you, but here's a suggestion: be confident about your new-found knowledge, see how far it takes you (hopefully in the right direction), but above all, have fun using it. You are now a bona fide expert in the art of bluffing about the world's oldest form of transport. Just put one foot in front of the other, aim towards the nearest country pub, and enjoy the scenery.

GLOSSARY

Bivvy bag A sleeping bag designed to be used in the open air. Looks like a coffin with a hole for your face – which helps emergency services with the identification process.

Bothy A mountain refuge, usually for more than two.

Breeches (also known as plus fours) Now only worn by hikers who might have strayed from the golf course.

Cairn A pile of stones typically marking a summit. Sometimes an artificial attempt to increase the height of a mountain.

Circular walk A successful walk where the hiker actually makes it back home again.

Corbett A mountain higher than 762m (2,500ft), but not as high as a Munro.

Cramp Your body's way of telling you to stop and admire the view.

Dilemma Finding two pubs next door to each other, and not knowing which one to go into first.

Fell walking The reason you have a grazed knee.

Gaiters Keep stones and water out of the tops of your boots, and the bottoms of your trousers unsoiled; more stylish than tucking your trousers into your socks.

Graham A mountain higher than 610m (2,000ft), but not as high as a Corbett or a Munro.

Hill A mound of earth that's not as high as a mountain.

Hillock A mound of earth that's not as high as a hill.

Ice axes Accessory to crampons.

JOGLE John o'Groats to Land's End (which is quicker than the other way round because it's downhill).

Kendal Mint Cake A mistake by a Kendal confectioner trying to make glacier mints. Eaten by Hillary and Tenzing at the summit of Everest in 1953. If it can help mountaineers conquer Everest, it can help you conquer that stile in front.

LEJOG Not French for jogging, but Land's End to John o'Groats.

Linear walk A route where the hiker is still at the pub and hasn't made it home yet.

Long Distance Walking Association For serious hikers.

Mountain A mound of earth higher than a hill.

Mountaineers and climbers Hard-core hikers with a death wish; keep out of their way.

Munro A mountain higher than 914.4m (3,000ft).

Munro-bagging A mission to climb the 282 Munros in Scotland; self-satisfied Munro-baggers are also known as windbags.

Pass What happens when a male and a female hiker try to use a kissing gate at the same time.

Pebble A mountain in Norfolk.

The Ramblers Self-help support group for people who can't give up hiking.

Rope Only to be used for skipping.

Shanks's pony Using one's legs as a means of transport (a method unknown to citizens of many American cities).

Tents If you can't afford a B&B or the YHA.

Triangulation pillar (also known as trig point). Proof that the Ordnance Survey team beat you to the summit.

Vibram Made in Italy but the BMW of boot soles.

Walking pole A hiker from Poland.

Youth hostels Cheap hikers' accommodation in outdoorsy areas mainly occupied by youths with an average age of 50.

A BIT MORE BLUFFING...

Available from all good bookshops

bluffers.com